Praise for *The De-Stress Effect*:

'Charlotte's book is my kind of read. I defy anyone to read this book and not relate it to their own life, see where there is room for improvement and, more importantly, use it to help alleviate that dreaded "stress" that enters all our lives! I love anything that does no harm, is noninvasive and can only do "good", and this book is that. Great advice, tips and help on how to really de-stress, and keep healthy and balanced in life. More importantly, it just makes sense. Good sense. I'm all for it!'
EMMA FORBES, TV AND RADIO PRESENTER

'Chronic stress affects everyone, depletes your mental and physical vitality and increases your risk of serious illness. The good news is that you can reverse its effects, and nurture resilience quickly and naturally. Charlotte beautifully brings together the science and traditions of nutritional, lifestyle and mind–body medicine in an immediately practical way so you can harness the 'De-Stress' effect and transform your life.'
BENJAMIN BROWN ND, THE BRITISH COLLEGE OF NUTRITION AND HEALTH AND AUTHOR OF *THE DIGESTIVE HEALTH SOLUTION*

'A great follow-up to The De-Stress Diet. Full of practical tips and advice, with a focus on mindful eating. Easy to read, powerful information for both your health and your weight.'
DR MARILYN GLENVILLE PhD, LEADING UK NUTRITIONIST SPECIALIZING IN WOMEN'S HEALTH AND AUTHOR OF *FAT AROUND THE MIDDLE*

'Charlotte simplifies a complex subject and gets straight to the point. She gives you pioneering techniques which are brilliant and no-nonsense. I can't recommend The De-Stress Effect highly enough.'
ANNIE ASHDOWN, AUTHOR OF *THE CONFIDENCE FACTOR* AND CO-HOST OF ITV 1'S, *KYLE'S ACADEMY*.

'The De-Stress Effect is brilliant, brilliant, brilliant. Personally, I think most people in the Western world would benefit from reading it! From cutting-edge, well-researched nutrition to simply-put science, balanced with yoga and mindfulness – this book will help the reader to get to the bottom of what type of stress they are suffering from, and offer simple yet effective solutions to help discover more health, well-being and calm.'
FIONA AGOMBAR, YOGA TEACHER AND AUTHOR OF *BEAT FATIGUE WITH YOGA*

'A truly holistic system for health, joy and wellbeing – easy to work through or dip into again and again to find ease within modern living. Charlotte deftly explains how to weave mindfulness into nutrition, yoga and exercise to create a rich experience and find out what really suits you.'
MARTIN CLARK, EDITOR OF *OM* MAGAZINE

'Charlotte's brilliant book is a gift for everyone suffering from all forms of stress. It explains why your body seems to be rebelling or burning out, and then shows you effective, practical approaches to get your life and health back on track.'

PHIL PARKER, EXPERT IN THE PSYCHOLOGY OF HEALTH HAPPINESS AND INVENTOR OF THE LIGHTNING PROCESS®

'With so much frequently conflicting and confusing information available about wellness and nutrition, it was a real pleasure to read Charlotte Watts's follow-up to The De-stress Diet and see her offering such clear advice on how to achieve wellness and calm in The De-Stress Effect. Solidly referenced and evidenced by sound science, you won't find any gimmicky or faddy advice here. Instead, it offers very clear guidelines to help you develop an effective stress-management toolkit, using exercise, yoga, mindfulness meditation and nutrition for different stress 'types' to find balance in a busy life. The morning and evening routines for introducing a less frenzied approach to your day are well worth exploring, and the principles for putting together healthy meals allow plenty of flexibility for different preferences and timescales. The yoga sequences are clearly illustrated and easy to follow, even for complete beginners. I will be recommending The De-Stress Effect to my coaching, yoga and nutrition clients.'

TRACY JOHNSON, YOGA TEACHER; INTEGRATIVE NUTRITION HEALTH COACH; CAREER, CONFIDENCE AND WELLNESS COACH

'Stress shuts us down: psychologically, emotionally and physically, cutting off our natural senses and killing our joy. Charlotte shows us how we can easily reconnect, and get refreshed, excited and back in our natural flow in really accessible and enjoyable ways.'

GEMINI ADAMS, AUTHOR OF THE FACEBOOK DIET: 50 FUNNY SIGNS OF FACEBOOK ADDICTION AND WAYS TO UNPLUG WITH A DIGITAL DETOX

'This is an invaluable book if you are a yoga practitioner, physical therapist or someone looking to find answers about why you are feeling the way you are. There is so much information out there now, but I believe that if you are going to buy one book that encapsulates everything you need to know – whether you are having recurrent health issues or physical injuries, or if you are stuck in a rut and just can't find an effective solution – then this is the book for you. It will support you from start to finish, and is an essential companion to understanding yourself and how you can make the right choices to create the life you want. I cannot recommend this book highly enough, which is why I insist that my clients, who are looking for long-term solutions, read it.'

GRAHAM STONES, DIRECTOR OF BROKEN YOGI AND FORMER NATIONAL KUNG-FU CHAMPION AND SPORTS INJURY THERAPIST FOR THE ENGLISH NATIONAL BALLET

THE
DE-STRESS
EFFECT

Rebalance Your Body's Systems for
Vibrant Health and Happiness

Charlotte Watts

HAY HOUSE

Carlsbad, California • New York City • London • Sydney
Johannesburg • Vancouver • Hong Kong • New Delhi

First published and distributed in the United Kingdom by:
Hay House UK Ltd, Astley House, 33 Notting Hill Gate, London W11 3JQ
Tel: +44 (0)20 3675 2450; Fax: +44 (0)20 3675 2451
www.hayhouse.co.uk

Published and distributed in the United States of America by:
Hay House Inc., PO Box 5100, Carlsbad, CA 92018-5100
Tel: (1) 760 431 7695 or (800) 654 5126
Fax: (1) 760 431 6948 or (800) 650 5115
www.hayhouse.com

Published and distributed in Australia by:
Hay House Australia Ltd, 18/36 Ralph St, Alexandria NSW 2015
Tel: (61) 2 9669 4299; Fax: (61) 2 9669 4144
www.hayhouse.com.au

Published and distributed in the Republic of South Africa by:
Hay House SA (Pty) Ltd, PO Box 990, Witkoppen 2068
Tel/Fax: (27) 11 467 8904; www.hayhouse.co.za

Published and distributed in India by:
Hay House Publishers India, Muskaan Complex, Plot No.3, B-2,
Vasant Kunj, New Delhi 110 070
Tel: (91) 11 4176 1620; Fax: (91) 11 4176 1630
www.hayhouse.co.in

Distributed in Canada by:
Raincoast Books, 2440 Viking Way, Richmond, B.C. V6V 1N2
Tel: (1) 604 448 7100; Fax: (1) 604 270 7161; www.raincoast.com

A significant portion of this book was originally published as
The De-Stress Diet (Hay House, 2012)

Text © Charlotte Watts, 2015

Yoga illustrations © Jackie Coulson, 2015

The moral rights of the author have been asserted.

The information given in this book should not be treated as a substitute
for professional medical advice; always consult a medical practitioner. Any
use of information in this book is at the reader's discretion and risk. Neither
the author nor the publisher can be held responsible for any loss, claim or
damage arising out of the use, or misuse, of the suggestions made, the failure
to take medical advice or for any material on third party websites.

A catalogue record for this book is available from the British Library.

ISBN: 978-1-78180-485-8

Printed and bound in Great Britain by TJ International Ltd, Padstow, Cornwall

Contents

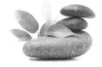

Introduction

Welcome to *The De-Stress Effect*, a highly practical manual that I hope you'll refer back to time and time again. It contains a multitude of suggestions to help you navigate your life's challenges and excitements in ways that work with and not against your body and mind. For over a decade, I've worked with clients suffering the effects of long-term and chronic stress, helping to alleviate their anxiety, insomnia, depression, Irritable Bowel Syndrome (IBS) and more. *The De-Stress Effect* presents the changes that have most resonated with those who needed a way back to health after living on 'constant alert'.

The book is a new incarnation of its predecessor, *The De-Stress Diet*, written with my co-author, journalist Anna Magee, as a result of our much-discussed interest in all things 'modern stress'. This stemmed from a consultation I did with Anna back in 2002, during which I said, 'Rather than think, "How do I look?", turn it around to ask "How do I feel?"'. As Anna has said since, considering the 'How do I feel?' question marked the start of a new relationship with her body and food, along with a new attitude, and you'll find that this question is a core part of the book.

The work I've done since *The De-Stress Diet* was written in 2011 has continued this 'feeling not thinking' personal and professional relationship with mind–body health. I've explored the roles that awareness in movement, stillness and being present play – not just in our lives, but also in how we approach nutrition.

Fast lives with high expectations shout 'fuel up!' to our bodies and our abundant worlds offer numerous possibilities to crave, grasp and want. Nowhere is this seen more acutely than in our relationship with food. The ancient survival mechanisms designed to give us the motivation to put in the hard work to find nourishment now struggle with too much choice and foods that play into quick-fix desires set off by stress.

Yes, we're up against a lot, but the routes to liberation are pretty enjoyable when we relax into them. I've been exploring how to meld these elements so that nutrition, body awareness, movement and meditation aren't just sitting in different boxes in our lives. Looking from a holistic angle, where they meet are the subtleties that can mean settling into healthy relationships with food and your body.

Many of us crave nature, vastness, expanse and space yet we feel conditioned to hem ourselves in with technology, speed, goal-orientation and self-criticism, imagining that a weekend away every so often will somehow redress the balance. This constrictive way of living is how the stress response has gained its negative connotation. Stress is seen as a judgement, a 'bad' state that needs to be fixed or cured.

This fits in nicely with a reductionist view of the world in which we break things down neatly into boxes, but it doesn't actually fit the definition of 'stress'. Stress is simply a provocation to a challenge, a call to act or react. The stress response is neither 'good' nor 'bad'; it's how it affects us *after* the event that determines whether we call it 'healthy' or 'unhealthy'. We'll explore this in more detail later in the book, and look at how adaptation and building resilience are key factors in transforming exhaustive stress into a positive challenge. We aren't looking to 'cure stress', but to reveal an attitude and lifestyle that allow body systems to have enough innate recovery capacity to absorb demands with grace.

From a young age, I felt overwhelmed by these stress responses. As a teenager, I felt isolated, depressed and deeply fatigued, finding relaxation and perspective very difficult to achieve. This followed me to art college, where I had a breakdown in the third year of my course, culminating in Chronic Fatigue Syndrome into my late twenties.

These patterns were always characterized by endless circles of painful Irritable Bowel Syndrome, migraines, depression, anxiety, panic attacks and insomnia, but those labels don't really sum up the experience for me. There was an abundance of fearful, tight-headed, self-defensive, jaw-clamping, eye-straining, gut-wrenching struggle that was difficult to describe, but in retrospect I can see this was driven by a heightened and continual stress response – especially as I've heard the same descriptions from many clients over the years.

Getting connected was a gradual process, one that led to the combination of elements featured in this book. Everything is presented here with the understanding that older wisdom needs to be applied to a modern context. I'm interested in the science (you'll find lots of it throughout, all meticulously referenced), but I'm also wary of letting the raging need to know, prove and categorize – which can be so reassuring – overtake our own *innate* knowing.

New neuroscience is revealing that our 'gut feelings' are true and should be listened to. What yogis call 'inner ears' and 'inner eyes' reside deep in the belly. Living neck up, in our heads, is really rather limiting, and more importantly, it cuts us off from feeling and living life to the full – evaluating when we could be experiencing. It can prevent us from tending to our foundational needs: what our bodies are communicating. If we use scientific information well, new research such as that into the beneficial effects of kindness, self-compassion and mindfulness can remind us that these simple attitudes are worth prioritizing, especially when our worlds might push them into the background.

If a symptom pops up, it's a message that something needs to be tended to, modified or given priority. Also, perhaps, that your body has been sending these messages for a while, but you've been too busy to listen. In our society we often tend to keep going, to 'push on through', medicate and suppress symptoms; we say, 'it's *just* stress' or simply ignore it as something minor. As modern medicine diagnoses disease states, and anything less may be dismissed, minor symptoms may be given the room to go unaddressed and grow into larger states of dis-ease.

I've experienced all seven of the 'Stress Suits' that I explore in chapter 5, and I'm now quite adept at recognizing the little signs that are gently knocking at the door, saying, 'Do you think you may be overdoing it?' Since I tend to take on too much, get excited and then feel a crash later, I've finally learned to have a little foresight when I start to crave sugar at 4 p.m., bloat around the belly and wake up feeling unrefreshed! This isn't being neurotic, just connected.

So why am I telling you all about me? Well, it's likely you can relate to some parts of my story if not others. Even if my travels are a world away from your own, they aren't alien. We're all human, all making our way through life as best we can, and given that you picked up this book, we have a shared interest in self-discovery and uncovering what best suits our true nature. Finding a flow, stride, rhythm or tune that feels mostly easier over mostly harder.

My skill lies in taking others through a transformative process that I hope to pass on to you in this book. Even at my lowest point, I still believed that change is always possible. I chose to find out how I could enjoy life more – alongside helping others to do the same – and I knew that would be an illuminating journey! The phrase 'keep doing what you do and you'll get what you got' resonated with me deeply and made me curious about how things could be different.

I've explored everything in these pages within my own life and still mix and match all the elements. I'm a born urbanite, which probably doesn't suit me, but I can't quite bring myself to move to the country. So I navigate within some imperfect variables and constantly play around with balance.

You may be able to relate to such a scenario. Like me, you may need a period of focusing inwards on change, and working out what makes you tick. This isn't to feed a self-obsessed, health-neurotic, navel-gazing mindset, but to find a new groove and eventually settle into the things that simply nurture good health and happiness without needing too much thought. A place where we know how to look after ourselves, know how to have a good time and know how to recover when we push the envelope – all with a smile and (mostly!) free of the inner critic.

I've given a six-week time frame for the nutritional changes you'll make as part of The De-Stress Effect – starting with De-Stress Eating Every Day in Part II. This isn't because six weeks is the time it takes to 'get better', but it is a good period to settle in new nutritional habits and have them feed out into every aspect of your life. This can create long-term change that sticks.

Even if entrenched symptoms like insomnia and depression take longer to recover fully from, the journey along the way can be one of the most rewarding you'll ever take. *The De-Stress Effect* is designed as an exploration into your body's natural wisdom – a way of listening to what it needs for you to live your life with ease, space and joy. Connecting with yourself helps you connect with others and with life.

There are loads of ideas in the book, but even if you just eat a little less sugar, walk a little bit more, sit on a park bench listening to the birds a little more often and laugh a whole lot more, you're going in the right direction.

Enjoy!

Charlotte x

PART I

Are You Stuck in the Stress Loop?

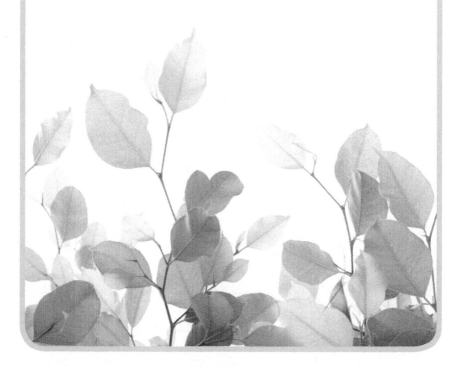

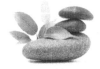

CHAPTER 1

Is Stress Ruling Your Life, Health and Happiness?

'He who knows others is wise, but he who knows himself is enlightened.'
LAO TZU

It's no secret that excess stress isn't healthy. This epidemic of the modern world is an underlying cause of low energy, anxiety, Irritable Bowel Syndrome (IBS), loss of sex drive, insomnia, depression, tooth-grinding, high blood pressure, skin problems, infertility, weight gain and gum disease.

In the UK, 12.8 million working days are lost to stress every year,[1] and 1.5 million people are dependent on benzodiazepines (highly addictive anti-anxiety drugs whose brand names include Ativan, Valium, Mogadon and Lbrium).[2] Although almost all of us complain about feeling stressed at work, one study found nearly a quarter of working people take no breaks and a third turn to comfort eating and extreme dieting to cope.[3]

With the World Health Organization estimating that by 2020, stress-related disorders will be the second leading cause of disabilities in the world, it's no wonder that the effects of stress, and how we manage them, are of great interest to researchers. Recent findings show that high levels of the stress hormone cortisol correlate with tendencies for major depression, cardiovascular disease, diabetes, autoimmunity and cancer, so we're beginning to understand that all aspects of our health have a relationship with stress.

If you chose to pick up this book, chances are you've recognized that things need to change and you're probably ready – or at least interested – to find other ways to cope with stress. If someone else gave you the book, you may or may not be ready to take its ideas on board. That's okay – we come to things when we're ready and even one simple change can have profound effects. So, let's see how life has been treating you.

THE STRESS GAUGE

How stressed are you *right now*? The questions below can be used as an indicator to check in and see how well you've been coping with those life challenges. You can come back to them regularly and use your responses – 'yes' or 'no' – to gauge whether stress has become overwhelming. In doing this, you can start to see patterns and notice the signs of excess stress before you reach breaking point.

Your behaviour

Do you:

- react to situations or events in a more dramatic or heightened way than you afterwards think you should have?

- feel overwhelmed if a task or demand you didn't expect occurs suddenly?

- feel demotivated, as if every chore is a bigger mountain than it was, say, a year ago?

- feel compelled to take on more and more, even if you don't think you can handle it?

- feel angry, scared, anxious or irritable – or swing from one to another?

- tend to take things on for others, regardless of your time limits and feelings?

- feel the need to 'just keep going' or to juggle all your balls in the air?

- avoid relaxing and letting go more and more?

- avoid difficult situations, people or crowds – even if you know, deep down, you might enjoy them?

- seek out exciting, high-risk situations, exercise or hobbies?

Stress is a heightened, excitatory response – galvanizing energy for the motivation and focus to get things done. Staying in this state can be overwhelming, with few dips in between to recover, gather in and come to rest.

How you feel

Do you:

- feel sensitive to bright lights, sudden noises and/or touch?

- feel unable to filter out different sounds in a room?

- feel less and less able to cope?

- want to hide from the world more and more?

- find yourself frowning, sighing or yawning often?

- find yourself snapping at people more and wishing you hadn't?

- feel upset more and more easily, at the slightest things?

- feel more vulnerable, fearful about the future or lacking in confidence?

- get less and less pleasure out of things you used to love?

- find small tasks harder and harder to complete?

Staying in the energetically intense state of stress means that we remain in a place of vigilance, which can become wearing. This can ultimately leave us too exhausted to do the activities that don't demand our attention loudly – like taking time for ourselves.

How you cope

Do you:

- use stimulants such as tea, coffee, cigarettes, alcohol, chocolate, sugar or recreational drugs as a 'fix' to keep you going or to ease the pressure?

5

- crave sugar, coffee, or the 'buzz' of achievement to feel alert and fulfilled?
- watch TV, play video games or surf the net as a way to switch off or numb?
- turn to behaviours such as excessive shopping, sex, drinking binges or arguments and find yourself relishing the drama or buzz?
- do large amounts of exercise – more than one hour in any one day or strenuous exercise on five or more days a week – with little rest?
- sink into phases – perhaps even entire weekends – of couch-potato slump?
- go through cycles of bingeing and overeating alternated with restricted diets?
- seem to get addicted to behaviours or substances more easily than you used to?
- feel compulsive about certain things – for example, cleaning, being organized, your iPhone or social networking habit – or have an excessive need to control the outcome of things at work?
- have a very low or exceedingly high appetite?

Continual stress has us living on a roller-coaster of energy and emotions, putting our seeking impulses on high alert to fuel up for food and, in the modern world, more 'stuff', because it's there. Highs and lows can become a way of life and we can yearn for balance and equanimity.

What's going on?

Do you:

- grind your teeth at night and/or clench your jaw during the day?
- have difficulty getting to sleep, or wake with a start in the small hours?
- find concentration, multi-tasking or remembering things more difficult than before?

- feel fuzzy, confused or disconnected?
- feel wired or on constant alert?
- experience sudden drops in energy, or constant fatigue?
- need to sleep more and more?
- feel unrefreshed on waking in the morning, or have to press the snooze button five times (at least) before getting up?
- get sick when you go on holiday, or catch every infection going?
- find yourself holding your breath or sighing unwittingly?

Keeping body mechanisms up in a continually excited zone is like running a car at 100 mph all the time. Crashes, wearing of parts and simply giving out become inevitable. Without allowing our nervous system to drop into full recovery state regularly, we're just making token pit stops and our bodies stay in a heightened, jangly state.

Your symptoms

Have you noticed:

- digestive issues such as bloating, belching or constipation?
- your skin breaking out or looking grey and dull, or the onset or flare-up of conditions such as eczema, acne or psoriasis?
- your skin is looking prematurely aged, greyish, or dehydrated around the cheeks and under your eyes?
- mood swings, feeling low or depressed?
- you're developing inflammatory conditions such as asthma, arthritis or hay fever?
- a tendency or sudden onset of allergies or food intolerances?
- increased headaches?
- excessive sweating or urination?
- reduced libido?
- heavy periods, PMS, menopausal or erectile problems?

Stress symptoms are a result of running everything too high, for too long. This translates across all body systems: digestive, immune, nervous, endocrine (hormonal) and so on. We'll explore how and why this happens and how to use these signals to listen and respond to your needs in a more connected and supportive way.

HOW STRESS AFFECTS YOUR BODY

Whatever your body and mind are expressing at the moment, you're living in the twenty-first century and unless you're on a remote island, you're likely to be subject to its constant streams of information and particular strain of demands. Sitting in a traffic jam, hearing the news that your four-year-old is ill at nursery, or dealing with a difficult boss are all examples of stressful everyday situations.

The term 'stress' refers to any physical, mental or emotional stimulus that provokes a reaction from the body. It can be caused by circumstances such as continual deadlines or sleepless nights with a baby, but it's also caused in more subtle ways by our underlying fears and worries – about losing our jobs, our homes, the people we love – things that affect our feelings of safety. The latter is something psychologists have termed 'psycho-social stress' and it's the most insidious, damaging kind.

You'll see your body referred to as 'mind–body' often in the book – a reminder that all parts of us are affected by every change and aspect of our lives, and that we can't separate out the emotional from the physical and vice versa.

Fight, flight or freeze: your body's stress response

Stress is a whole mind–body response. Every time you're under any type of stress, your body will activate its immediate stress response in exactly the same way. This is a survival mechanism that evolved in humans over millions of years and there's little you can do to escape it. Whatever the crisis, person or situation, a complex cascade of hormonal, neurological and physical processes is set in motion in the brain and body, known as the *stress response*.

We still play out this reaction, set in our biological programming from the days when our ancestors had sabre-toothed tigers forcing them to 'fight, flee or freeze'. Each time you face a stressful situation – bad boss, marriage crisis or traffic jam – your body reacts as though it's life-threatening and kicks in its response to fight through the danger, run away from it or become immobilized and static.

Your stressor never relents (you never slay the tiger because the tiger is your job and it's always, well, *there*), so the same whole mind–body process keeps jackpotting over and over, and that's when the damage occurs. You can't override this primal response, but you can help your reactions lessen and become more appropriate to the true level of danger.

Down at the biological level

When we sense something stressful, our hormones immediately send a cascade down from the brain to the adrenal glands through a route called the HPAA (hypothalamic-pituitary-adrenal axis) to release adrenaline, increasing our heart rate and sending blood coursing around our muscles for that ready-for-anything feeling. If the brain perceives the stress continuing beyond the time the adrenaline is 'needed' (you're still in the midst of that deadline), it moves to plan B.

Adrenaline works for up to an hour before it's reabsorbed, but if your body senses the need to keep up a heightened response, the hypothalamus deep in your brain secretes corticotropin-releasing hormone (CRH). This then signals the pituitary gland at the base of your brain to release adrenocorticotropic hormone (ACTH) into the bloodstream. Then, ACTH tells the adrenal glands to release the major stress hormone, cortisol.[4]

Cortisol is a steroid hormone, made from fat, and we always need some running around our systems, governing our energy levels and metabolic rate. Ideally it's at high levels in the morning to get us up and at low levels at night to allow sleep; continual stress often means evening highs that get in the way of our dropping off to sleep or enjoying good-quality sleep when we do. Adrenaline is a protein hormone, only released in a reactive way when needed for perceived danger. Like adrenaline, cortisol has a purpose when we're stressed and small amounts provide short bursts of energy, focus and increased sensory sensitivity.

9

The cortisol-weight connection

Cortisol stimulates appetite[5] for fuel during periods of prolonged stress and its overproduction turns those extra calories into fat. Cells in the abdomen have more receptors for cortisol than any other part of the body, so most of that fat gets stored around the tummy.[6,7] People who produce excess cortisol tend to have bulky waistlines and apple-shaped bodies rather than pear-shaped ones, but weight can be affected in other ways.

Chronically elevated cortisol can lead to loss of muscle tone[8] and inhibit thyroid function,[9] slowing metabolic rate and making weight loss difficult. Research from Harvard Medical School in the USA surveyed over 2,500 men and women aged between 25 and 74 and found that weight for the men was most closely associated with job-related demands, financial difficulties and a low support network. For the women, along with job and money problems, strained relationships were the major contributor.[10]

THE STAGES OF STRESS

In the 1930s, Hungarian endocrinologist Hans Selye studied what happens to the body under short- and long-term pressure. He described the body's reactions as a three-stage process:

Stage one: alarm

This is our immediate reaction to the stressor – adrenaline-fuelled fight, flight or freeze – and in the short term it causes an immune system boost, both to activate inflammation to stop us bleeding to death if wounded (remember, the body is thinking 'sabre-toothed tiger') and to fight off possible infections of said wound.

Today, 'fighting' might mean severe tetchiness or outbursts, and 'flight' walking out on an argument, social withdrawal, numbing with alcohol or sugar or watching TV in order to 'switch off'. 'Freeze' can mean complete shut-down – no eye contact and a thousand-yard stare – often a result of past trauma in the mix.

Stage two: resistance

As a stressful situation continues, physical processes happen to help us adapt. Take extended pressure at work – under increased mental demands, the body will instinctively release more stress hormones to help us stay focused. Meanwhile the immune system is suppressed, sparing energy for the tasks at hand.

Stage three: chronic stress

When stressful situations continue for more than a few weeks, the body, which began by resisting the stress with gusto, begins to lose its adaptive capacity. This will manifest differently in different people (see Stress Suits in chapter 5).

The immune system may get stuck in inflammatory mode, leading to stress-related skin, joint and/or digestive problems while the body's ability to fight invading bacteria or viruses is chronically suppressed. Continual sore throats, sniffles or cold sores are warning signs. People with long-term stress may succumb to severe infections, autoimmune conditions, increased blood pressure and heart attacks due to this poor *immune modulation*.[11]

REROUTING AND RESENSITIZING

Fight or flight mode directs blood flow away from the extremities and towards the heart, lungs, legs and back to help maximize running and fighting power (yes, even if you just get an upsetting text), creating tension there and reducing fine motor skills dramatically. In the long term, this can cause loss of interoception, the ability to feel the subtleties of our inner body as bigger physical actions are prioritized. This is one reason that a body awareness practice like yoga can help us reconnect and come down out of stress modes.

This rerouting of circulation by stress affects many systems. It diverts blood and energy away from sexual function – not crucial under the threat of attack – and is a common cause of low libido and erectile dysfunction as well as being linked to infertility. Stress halts digestion, meaning food left undigested can cause nausea, add to constipation or even cause a reflex for ejection by vomiting or diarrhoea.

Have you ever noticed that a frightened animal urinates before running? That contraction of the bladder helps to 'lighten the load', so a common stress sign is frequent urination.

Within the field of psychoneuroimmunology it's theorized that modern stressors are directed towards our guts and brain, leaving our immune system barely aware of the skin and others body parts on the periphery. Skin conditions that persist could well be the immune system simply not noticing them. After all, the skin's first design was for protection from outside forces, not inner stress. Moving away from modern brain chatter to regular contact with the forces of nature ('good stress', see page 46) has been shown to support immune modulation.

THE GUT–BRAIN CONNECTION

Much stress research has been directed towards the gut, where the *enteric nervous system* (ENS, aka 'The Second Brain') is a complex mass of nerve cells running the entire length of your digestive tract, from mouth to anus. About the size of a cat's brain, it can operate separately to the central nervous system (brain and spinal cord) but is in continual dialogue with the brain.

With research now showing that 90 per cent of information flows from gut to brain and only 10 per cent 'top-down', simply attempting to soothe ourselves by talking to the mind and staying up in our heads can only get us so far. Talking therapies are essential for those who need to articulate feelings and make sense of situations, but if we neglect a whole-body self-care approach alongside, we can't expect our nervous systems to *truly believe* that we're safe and let go of the need to react as if we're under constant threat.

Trusting our 'gut feelings'

Research is helping us to understand that the ENS plays a part in our mental and emotional states, but not cognitive decision-making or conscious thoughts, so it is at the heart of *intuitive* decisions.[12] A group of peptides (proteins) called corticotropin-releasing factors (CRF) coordinate stress responses and have a direct effect on the gut. They can create inflammation, weaken the gut wall, contribution to hypersensitivity, increase pain perception and change the movement of digestive muscle.

These felt responses can be remembered and used to assess the relative safety of a new situation compared to a previous one. So, say you felt unsafe on a particular train journey, the next time you board a train your gut feelings remind your brain that it needs to be alert for danger and you might feel uneasy.

When past or present trauma, grief, job stress, lack of support or unreliable living conditions tell your brain (via your gut) that the world is an unsafe place to live, this can create a state often described by my clients as 'constant alert'. Here we can find ourselves stressed by the smallest things, with sensitivity to noise and light and wanting to hide away sure signs that we're stuck on high alert.

Heightened senses are there to keep us aware of possible danger, but this is a different 'awareness' to the one we'll explore later, within the chapters on mindfulness. This is more about 'beware' – our eyes and ears letting in continual information without discernment – and it makes being in crowds overwhelming. It can be difficult to focus on just one person talking in a crowd and filter out peripheral sights and sounds.

Our gut feelings are on protective overdrive and our HPAA is prompted over and over again to 'keep reacting!', often telling us to 'just get out of there'. Does that sound exhausting? It is, on all levels, and as well as physical fatigue, it makes the energy needed to express emotions around other people seem a bridge too far.

ADRENAL FATIGUE – DOES IT EXIST?

Your doctor may not acknowledge the term 'adrenal fatigue', one used in natural health circles to describe a state in which our adrenal glands have been pumping out stress hormones for so long that they become depleted. Stress hormones aren't all bad: we need them to get going and if they're on a go-slow, our ability to feel motivated and energetic becomes dampened.

However, medical opinion is beginning to accept adrenal fatigue; a recent meta-analysis of research papers on 'burnout' acknowledged that this physical or mental collapse was characterized by lowered cortisol (particularly on rising) and the stress hormone DHEA (see page 49).

Burnout falls outside the category of a 'true' disease and is often medically treated as depression or not at all, even though the evidence shows it's associated with coronary disease and heart attacks. In a 2013 paper titled *The Medical Perspective on Burnout*, lowered response of the HPAA was shown, meaning that after a period of overactivity, the response can dampen and shut down – leaving us feeling unresponsive, listless and unable to get going.[13] This can even stop us having appropriate reactions to circumstances we *should* be registering as stressful – like not studying for an exam or finding a better job.[14]

Low morning cortisol can stop us being enthused for the day ahead[15] – we may turn to caffeine and sugary breakfasts to get us out of the door. Hitting the snooze button right up to the limit is a sign that stress may have worn you down.

Avoiding or recovering from burnout

This level of fatigue needs support for the adrenal glands and hormonal, nervous, digestive, immune and other symptomatic body systems when stress throws off our ability to adapt and recover.[16] It's unsustainable to keep up stress and expect that just pumping out energy will be okay without recharging the batteries. To prevent exhaustion and worsening of stress-related conditions, we need to reset and allow all systems to recognize the resting place they need to routinely come back to.

If not, burnout could be looming on the horizon. I say this not to stress you further, but to impress on you that now is the time to treat yourself well. If you're feeling that you've reached or are nearing system shut-down, be assured there is a way back, but it does take a change in mindset.

New pathways

We always have a choice to change and if previous attitudes, habits and lifestyle have got you to this place, it's important to recognize that something has to give. Too much of anything – partying, working, parenting and looking after others over yourself – is an imbalance. With this book you can explore how to find new ways of living with the self-care you need to rebuild depleted resources.

This can be one of the most illuminating and rewarding journeys you'll make; those who have come back from burnout or a 'nervous breakdown' often feel enormous gratitude that it allowed them to shift their lives to a more enjoyable pace, openness and direction. It isn't always plain sailing, but we can learn how to ride the rough waves with more ease.

If we start listening to our body's needs, it won't have to take back the reins and let us know that 'enough is enough' by enforcing shut-down and going into 'conservation mode'. Let's now explore ways to let your body and mind know they are being tended to and loved, so you can feel safer at a deeper, gut level. Then your whole system can relax and your symptoms start to decrease. Letting your mind rest and your body heal is a good place to start.

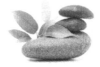

CHAPTER 2

De-Stress for Improved Quality of Life

'If you have built castles in the air, your work need not be lost... Now put foundations under them.'
HENRI DAVID THOREAU

The De-Stress Effect helps you find the space and self-care to truly feel what's right for you – intuitively and from an open-minded outlook. Stress takes us away from this state, towards responses designed to simply deal with immediate threat, where we often feel 'locked in' and treat ourselves harshly just to keep going.

Stress has us acting from a fear-based and therefore negative outlook, so fostering a sense of safety through kind attention can help draw us round to seeing things more positively. This is where we turn our focus inwards and notice how we're feeling, with a sense of care and compassion.

One of the most accessible, free and well-researched routes to lowered cortisol is mindfulness and meditation, where this compassion is at the core. In the Shamatha Project,[1] a comprehensive, long-term control-group study of the effects of meditation training on mind and body supported by the Dalai Lama, participants engaged in attentional skills such as mindfulness of breathing, observing mental events and cultivating loving-kindness, compassion and empathic joy over a three-month period.

One of the study's researchers, Tonya Jacobs, said that 'The more a person reported directing their cognitive resources to immediate sensory experience and the task at hand, the lower their resting cortisol.'

That is why the practice of mindfulness is woven throughout all the practical suggestions in this book: bringing sensory attention to our relationships with food, lifestyle and movement can play a part in helping us feel connected and safe. This then creates cortisol-lowering De-Stress loops (see chapter 4), in which we gravitate towards those choices and activities that feed a contented and positive view of life.[2]

Mindfulness is the practice of being fully present and feeling 'what is' without judgement – whether that's while you eat, during a conversation, at a work meeting, in a yoga pose or as you're washing the dishes. We can 'drop in', notice how we feel and simply make the choice to be present in one or two breaths. This is the state from where we make more reflective and less impulsive decisions – and change can stick.

Don't worry too much about what mindfulness means. It simply refers to the quality of focus and attention we bring to each moment. However, that can sound pretty abstract, as it's all about experience. We can't *think* our way to feel; in fact, analysis and description just get in the way. In chapter 3 (Enjoy Each Moment) and chapter 15 (The Mindfulness Practices), there are plenty of simple ways to cultivate your mind and body's habits towards meeting the world with more ease and less stress.

Throughout the book you'll see mindfulness referred to in various ways – awareness, attention, self-compassion, presence, consciousness, connection, attunement and yoga. These all refer to the intention to 'be awake' during as many moments of our lives as possible and to drop into the stride that's naturally set for us. Much stress and unhappiness is caused by pushing against what we need: in Western cultures, decision-making from the head rather than the heart (or belly) is lauded – thinking over feeling; objective over subjective – and this conditioning can stop us listening to what our bodies are trying to tell us. Western medicine works to suppress symptoms of stress, but pay attention and you can get to the root causes and break the cravings, discontent, dis-ease and mind chatter that stress feeds.

Adopting a viewpoint of kind attention moves our habitual language away from the often used 'fighting' or 'combatting' stress. Using more compassionate and considered (rather than stressful and combative) language – words like 'relieving' or 'releasing' – helps us be as caring and gentle with ourselves as we would with others.

THE DE-STRESS EFFECT PRINCIPLES

Curiosity and exploration are necessary for true change to occur. Quick fixes or short-term regimens simply don't work, but flooding your day-to-day life with attitudes and applications that you can play around with creates fun and nurture – and it just feels right.

1. 'How do I feel?'

Our culture places so much emphasis on *external* factors, from gauging health by outside appearance to comparing ourselves to the bendy student on the next yoga mat. This outside focus clouds the real truth: that all of those projections are subjective and deciding our world view on how attractive/thin/successful/popular we perceive ourselves to be at any given time limits us and can't make us happy.

Moving inwards to how we *feel* – and listening to our bodies rather than the constant barrage of thoughts – is the way to contentment. Even if the answer to the question 'How do I feel?' isn't always 'Great!', *this* is the essence of mindfulness. Throughout this book, diet and lifestyle changes are offered to help you feel the best you can be – and to feel more acceptance when that's not so good.

This is the optimal starting place to recognize and explore the most effective strategies for you to escape from stress and sensory overload, or just to gather in to a place of perspective whenever you need to. With chronic stress or trauma, our ability to feel can often become numbed, so the practices in chapter 16 (Yoga as Awareness) are designed to help us connect back to feeling. The mindfulness practices throughout the book will help meet any locked in stresses coming out that may feel overwhelming.

2. Treat yourself as a friend

The awareness that we foster by asking 'How do I feel?' needs fertile ground to enable it to liberate us from the stress of constant brain chatter and negative thoughts. Self-compassion is the quality that allows us to move through change and meet responses with openness. Exploration means that some things will resonate with you and others will not. Be prepared to let things go and try something else – this isn't a failing on your part but a way to find out what *does* suit you; this is important information.

If you've ever tried to set new habits but been set back by self-criticism or judgement when things aren't 'perfect', now is the time to stop giving yourself such a hard time. There is no 'one size fits all' answer and holding on to that rigid outlook or any standards of perfection (no such thing) are a recipe for creating the kind of poor self-worth spiral that has us self-medicating on chocolate (again).

Kind attention and speaking to ourselves with the tones and words we'd use towards someone we love can be the difference between hours of guilt about that chocolate bar or truly enjoying it – having the space to notice how it made you feel, learning from that and moving on. If you're in the habit of looking after others' needs over your own, self-compassion is what's needed now.

3. Pleasure matters

It's the rich sense memories that come from feeling better – not extreme diets or regimens – that make people stick with healthy lifestyles. Sense memories are the clear associations between change and feeling better that our bodies remember – and these give us both reasons and motivation to keep it up.

The De-Stress Effect is a complete programme with not only physical but also emotional benefits, bringing you a powerful sensory reason to stick with it long term – *and* you'll see knock-on results in the way you look. Ultimately, this is about living as Nature intended – with plenty of sunlight, touch, healthy sex, laughter, movement and high-quality food – to reach our highest levels of stress-free, pleasurable health success.

4. Find your rhythm with food

In the modern world, we have a huge amount of choice, but this can create conflict and stress. Nowhere is this seen more than in our relationships with food. This was once a resource that was hard to find, with the only choice presented there and then, but today we have to make constant decisions about what to eat, often combined with the continual struggle of 'what we want' vs 'what we need'.

Stress creates the survival urge to seek energy for quick responses – it tells us that we 'need' that cake – while our more rational inner dialogue can pipe up with a stress-provoking and guilt-ridden lecture on healthy eating. When our bodies simply react in the way they're designed to, an abundance of choice can have us trapped in problematic relationships with sugar, refined carbohydrates and junk fats.

Providing your body with the nourishment it needs for energy, mood and appetite control has a chicken-and-egg effect – it lets your body know it has sustainable fuel for any eventuality and the satisfaction this creates lessens the frequency and magnitude of cravings. Honouring the way our Stone Age ancestors ate with a dose of reality for twenty-first-century living can have you naturally attracted to the foods that best support you and liberated from the constant inner dialogue about what is 'good' or 'bad' (see chapter 6).

5. Know yourself

When stress is long-term and chronic, a variety of symptoms develop, depending on body make-up. One person might have an acne breakout while another becomes hyper-manic. In chapter 5, you can discover which 'Stress Suit' you're wearing at any given time and how to help your own tendencies. Through this increased self-awareness you'll discover the fundamental lifestyle and diet principles that work for you – not your friend, partner or 'informed' work colleague – by feeling their effects and setting a long-term rhythm in place.

6. Some stress is good

Not all stress is bad; the right kind can have a positive effect on the body, allowing us to build healthy resources to react with flexibility rather than knee-jerk responses that create more stress. This isn't always about being comfortable, though: stepping out of your comfort zone and actively seeking healthy stressors can create adaptability and resilience. This is where mindfulness becomes most important; learning to be with all sensations – comfortable and not-so-much – can free us from the constant stress-producing dialogue about whether we like stuff or not. And yes, this is being kind to yourself!

7. Lay the foundation

Reclaiming your mornings, and how you set the tone for the day, gives you strong roots to connect back to. A nutritious, protein-based breakfast and a more spacious start allow your body to find the natural rhythm it needs to become stronger and more able to cope with your daily demands. With this come optimal energy and appetite patterns, freedom from food obsessions and stepping away from the urge to snack. This is explored in more depth in chapter 11 (A Morning Revolution).

8. Live naturally

You don't have to exercise to exhaustion to get the body and mood benefits of exercise. De-Stress Effect movement is about increased everyday activity. The yoga chapter guides you to connect with your daily body expressions and release the tensions that stress may have caused.

The movement/exercise chapter then harnesses the growing interest in primal fitness in sports science, encouraging you to integrate natural, varied movement into your everyday life. Walking, swimming, strength training and/or team sports, along with regular, de-stressing yoga, will get you feeling – and looking – great and better able to deal with the stressors in your life, creating as well as using up energy.

9. Rest, not just sleep

One of the most important aspects of The De-Stress Effect is rest. Hunter-gatherers would have had high-activity days followed by low-activity days. This would have reduced the likelihood of crippling injuries, preserved precious (yes, *precious*!) calories and given the body a chance to recharge itself.

Yet in the modern world we go on and on and on, with less sleep and rest than we need and then wonder why we're tired. Finding space in our hyper-connected, oversubscribed lives – even if only for a few moments a day – to do nothing, take some conscious breaths or simply feel our feet on the ground is essential to this plan.

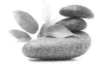

CHAPTER 3

Enjoy Each Moment

*'In the end, only three things matter: how much you
loved, how gently you lived, and how gracefully
you let go of things not meant for you.'*
THE BUDDHA

In the West, the Buddhist practice of mindfulness has increased in popularity in the last few decades, meeting the awareness that we're becoming more and more distracted from our feelings, our natural rhythms and our compassion to ourselves and others – the root of our psycho-social stress. Mindfulness is practised as a specific type of meditation, or as being attuned to the present moment at any given time.

It's also an intrinsic part of a yoga practice or meditative movement like T'ai chi, where we stay conscious of sensations arising from the body (interoception), and can be brought to any movement we do. Here's a definition of mindfulness to start from, but true understanding comes from simply trying and not worrying too much about the outcome:

*Mindfulness is the specific practice of paying attention
to our 'present moment' experience with an open and
curious mind – with compassion and no judgement.*

As Jon Kabat-Zinn – who was instrumental in bringing mindfulness to a Western audience – says: 'The practice of mindfulness... is living your life

25

as if it really mattered from moment to moment. The real practice is life itself.' His book *Full Catastrophe Living* takes its title from the film *Zorba the Greek*, in which the titular character says he has 'wife, house, kids, everything... the full catastrophe'.

This isn't said negatively, but with joy for the whole cascade of experience that life brings. When stress has us hiding from the full spectrum, bringing a quality of attentiveness to how we move through the day can allow us to live fully and adapt to changes as they arise.

Every tweak to our environmental habits (diet, movement, relaxation, living conditions) prompts a period of biochemical and behavioural shift. We're designed to continually adapt to these; this *allostasis* is the constant response to come back to balance (*homeostasis*), but as Kabat-Zinn says, its capacity can be worn down by stress if we don't learn how to ride the '*sorrows, dilemmas, tragedies and ironies*'.

GROOVY NEW BRAIN

In the last 15 years or so, new brain-imaging techniques have allowed scientists to map our brain and nervous system responses, showing that different parts of the brain can grow or shrink according to use. Contrary to previous thought, we now know that we can build new neural pathways (yes, old dogs *can* learn new tricks!) and change the ways we perceive and respond to the world around us.

Replacing old grooves with new habits isn't only possible, it keeps our brain active, engaged and sprightly. Getting stuck in a rut creates a non-adaptive stress of its own and often results in fear of change or a lack of enthusiasm to try new things. We respond massively to expectation – as seen in the placebo effect – so if we *believe* things can't change, then they don't. If we're simply open to trying new things, we're creating our own new landscapes through neural change – which is very exciting!

How can each moment be enjoyable?

This chapter is called Enjoy Each Moment not to add an expectation of perfection; real life isn't a world of perpetual rainbows (scary) and feeling sadness is vital to being able to feel joy. Mindfulness is about accepting things as they are, right now, recognizing that they always change and moving our perception from labelling experience as good/bad/neutral. It's the understanding that *all* experience is equally valid and important – even a heightened stress response is telling us something – we just need to be listening to what that might be.

As the thirteenth-century Persian mystic Rumi said of negative thoughts and feelings in his poem *The Guest House* '…they may be clearing you out for some new delight'. The one thing we can be certain of is that everything changes, so we let it all come and let it all go. The enjoyment comes from being able to simply be, with this flux as proof that we're alive! If we dare to see all experience through fresh, new eyes and step away from the ego-driven 'I know', we can feel each moment is brand new and get a whole lot more out of life.

New science for old wisdom

Tonya Jacobs, of the aforementioned Shamantha Project, says that 'people who dwell on painful past memories, or who develop anxiety about their future, typically have higher stress levels'. She adds that 'the idea that we can train our minds in a way that fosters healthy mental habits, and that these habits may be reflected in mind–body relations, isn't new; it's been around for thousands of years across various cultures and ideologies, [but it] is just beginning to be integrated into Western medicine as objective evidence accumulates.'

Practice: simply be

The way to experience mindfulness is simply to try it. This isn't unfamiliar; in fact, you do it all the time, but maybe not consciously. It's where you might feel 'at one' with your body and your surroundings. Try sitting in a familiar place – on your sofa, on a park bench or in a café – and when you might usually start looking at your phone or thinking about 'stuff', instead really *be* where you are at that point in time.

Feel body sensations, hear noises and see sights as they are – and as they change from moment to moment. Watch when you wander off and draw yourself back to your changing perceptions, without the need to comment, analyse or evaluate. Simply feel.

You don't have to be perfect

By dropping into the present moment and making space you'll start to see that your body wants to be calmer, less agitated and more connected to the world and the people around you. It's not that mindfulness is a relaxation system; it's not a practice of solving anything.

We know that life is stressful and we're not working from the premise that you're imperfect and need fixing, but a by-product of stepping back from reactivity is noticing that our bodies are always looking to come back to rest and to conserve energy. They are wired to calm down as soon as we let them – it's just that so often our busy lives and minds get in the way of this happening.

Moving away from distraction

The nature of our lives and minds is faster and more stressful than ever. To find peace, space and calm takes effort, dedication to consistent practice and for many of us, scheduling in to nestle between the ever-growing distractions that could fill our time. We live in a culture that celebrates 'doing' and doing that fast and with more of it. Yet all of this achieving and hitting goals is an avoidance of simply 'being'.

It's much easier for those of us with busy brains to make a new list than it is to shut off our smartphones and walk away from the TV. Continually giving and receiving information is stealing from ourselves, though; thinking over feeling, brain over body is a constantly stressful energy output and our bodies are relieved when our fuel-guzzling big brains finally rest.

Practice: letting go

Noticing what we're holding on to and what's ready to leave is a flow that we can drop into through a mindfulness practice. It's very human to want to hold on to thoughts and evaluations, as we can often believe that these make up who we are. Being open to change takes trust that our brain chatter isn't 'us'. Try writing down everything you think for 10 minutes and you'll soon see that there's an awful lot of noise! Letting go doesn't mean losing ourselves, but it does mean releasing things that no longer serve us and being open to more rewarding patterns.

A NEW RELATIONSHIP WITH TIME

The quality of the time we have depends on how much we're really there. So often we are off somewhere else, musing and ruminating on the past or planning and projecting into the future. To be still, in the present and truly noticing it without the need to change, judge or comment is a skill that often gets buffeted away by the noise and velocity of other distractions.

Being still, quiet and even slow are qualities that are often less appreciated in our culture; 'less is more' is often a novel concept and there are tendencies to miss the more subtle and rich moments when we're quickly rushing through to the next.

It can even seem uncomfortable to be silent and still after noise and bustle, but the more we become accustomed to quiet, the less we feel the need to fill it. You know that 'uncomfortable silence' you can have while sitting with someone in a car or over lunch? Rather than feeling the need to fill the gap, simply being with and feeling another person's presence can allow you to feel a whole lot more connected to them.

When we truly turn up to the moment, we can notice that time seems to fly. We drop into meditative alpha brainwaves (shown to reduce cortisol) whenever we become truly absorbed in the moment – for example, while gardening, knitting, painting or playing golf – but also allowing ourselves to be 'bored' and with time itself.

Expanse over contraction

Stress has a contracting effect; we physically and mentally recoil from the shock, hardening and shutting down to protect ourselves in the first instance. Over the next few breaths, if we can stay in the moment and recognize that the stress isn't actually life-threatening, we have the choice to allow ourselves to expand, soften and release the tension accumulated, even shaking it off if need be.

It can help when either meditating or in the face of events, words or situations that make you feel 'locked in', to gather courage with the inhalation and use it to feel an expanding out through your whole being with the exhalation. In this way we can soften our outer shell and feel awareness rather than self-defence as we meet the world. Soon we can begin to accept that it's actually more self-protective to stay pliable and intuitive than hardened and reactive and we can become calmer in the face of stressors.

Body awareness

Our top-heavy, brain-led culture can have us cut off from the neck down and feeling that our mind is the centre of our being. When our thoughts become dominant we can lose connection with what our body is trying to tell us (for example, 'go to bed earlier!') and start to over-identify with the voices in our head.

If you've ever had that feeling that you're narrating your life inside your head, it's time to give the voices a rest. Choosing to step aside from our internal dialogue and focus on our bodily sensations can help redirect focus. In this way, we can navigate change by really experiencing new tastes, movement patterns and challenges – we don't actually need to judge and decide if we deem them 'good' or 'bad' but rather give them time and patience to settle in.

Self-compassion isn't just positive thinking

Being 'present' asks us to meet things that may feel uncomfortable, unsettling, upsetting or even painful. Creating an expanse in which

30

anything that comes up has room to move, change and even be let go of, also makes room for self-compassion or *heartfulness*. As the wonderful mindfulness teacher Cathy-Mae Karelse says, *'Compassion is not fluffy'* – it takes courage and staying power to hold whatever comes up and be with it.

Although it's good to be positive, forcing the issue can cause a rebound effect. Our subconscious looks out for our best survival interests because it evolved at a time when we had to assume that a noise in the forest could well be a threat. This inbuilt fear response to our negative inner voice is still part of our make-up today and like any voice it wants to be heard. So when fearful warnings pop into your head, first listen and let your subconscious know you aren't ignoring it. Then thank it for its continued vigilance for your safety, but offer that you've found another strategy and breathe into your heart, putting a hand there if it helps.

This is also true for cravings: if we can *be* with these primal responses and not just numb them with food (or other substances), we can start to feel there may be other options available. This is further discussed in chapter 7 and the loving-kindness meditation on page 189 helps create kinder new grooves. A recent study of female students showed that even three weeks of this self-compassion practice improved resilience.[1]

MINDFULNESS ANYWHERE

My hope here is to give you permission to find meditation and mindfulness, however and wherever suits you. You can meditate formally (see chapter 15) or be completely present while doing a simple repetitive activity such as ironing, gardening or stuffing envelopes, with no background stimulus from the TV, radio and so on.

'As soon as you honour the present moment, all unhappiness and struggle dissolve, and life begins to flow with joy and ease.'
ECKHART TOLLE

You can actively watch your breath, shoulders and jaw release as you simply take a few moments to stop and pause. Many people find activities such as swimming or walking meditative, and they are great ways of optimizing the free time you have to both move and relax – with no iPad or phone calls to distract you or stimulate your mind. Sitting on a park bench for a few minutes or putting your phone away on the train is a vast improvement on never finding any time for centring yourself.

Mindful daily living

Regularly 'checking in' to meet ourselves can help us:

- Connect with our more primal selves to actually notice what's going on around us, rather than rushing past.

- Connect with our intuition and instinct to feel, rather than thinking about what any given situation requires.

- Find refuges – places and situations where we feel safe, calm and supported. Stress and the anxiety it creates mostly come from a deep-seated sense of 'not safe'.

- Accept that good things and bad things happen, but we learn, let go and move on.

- Look for opportunities to feel joy, ease and peace in our lives and in our relationships with others.

- Make food and lifestyle changes with a view to long-term change that will stick.

- Practice gratitude for the good things we have, rather than focusing on the negative.

- Notice those activities that help to reduce some of the stress effects identified in the Stress Gauge on pages 4–7.

Practice: find mindful peace amid all the noise

1. Continually look at the world around you, noticing the little details of trees, buildings, situations, etc., helps to bring you out of the constant noise of your head.

2.   De-clutter your environment (desk, bedroom, cupboards) and therefore your mind – having lots of stuff just serves to keep us feeling locked in and disengaged.

3.   If work seems overwhelming, step away from tasks that are creating stress and do something mundane and simple that 'needs doing'. Filing, tidying or organizing can switch brain mode and have a meditative quality.

4.   Find a bit of space daily – we can get into the trap of waiting until holidays or weekends to relax, but our bodies and minds need to restore continually and life is to be lived now. Try sitting on a bench in the sun, lying in the bath, or anything else that encourages you to stop and gather in. Look for the space between thoughts.

5.   Talk less and listen more: don't just wait for your turn to speak.

6.   Try not to complain or gossip: look at the intention behind your words and the seeds you sow.

Slowing down

We live in a fast-paced culture where speed of execution is valued and praised. While this can get much done, we run the risk of becoming attached to doing too much and exhausted in the process. If we deliberately slow down our tasks or actions we can begin to notice all of our senses feeding back the minutiae of our experience. Try the Mindful Eating exercise on page 93.

Every action has the potential for a meditative quality when we aren't experiencing fear or anger. Bringing a sense of compassion and gratitude to the execution of a simple task can help it become less 'driven' left-brain based and more 'creative and feeling' right-brain focused, where you can help regulate fear-based responses. As you move through your days, you can slow down some of the actions you do automatically and cultivate patience. For example:

•   Washing the dishes, opening your mail, watering the plants… watch out for when you 'go through the motions'.

- Cleaning your teeth or moisturizing your face – for body contact and self-care.

- Walking down the street, choosing groceries – our public actions can also involve speech and interactions with others where we can notice how we might rush to react, offer unwanted opinions or jump to conclusions when we don't allow time and space in communications.

Taking it forward

In the next chapter we'll explore the human relationship with stress, mind–body and food. Learning how we got to where we are always runs the risk of sending the vigilant and analytical side of our brains working overtime to deconstruct. If you feel you haven't been looking after yourself well, please don't waste energy dissecting past habits with judgement. Information has the power to help us understand ourselves and move forward with a new perspective.

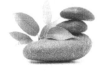

CHAPTER 4

How Stress Creates Loops

'The best time to plant a seed was 20 years
ago. The second best time is now.'
<small>CHINESE PROVERB</small>

Stress isn't all in your head – it sends waves throughout your entire being and out into your life. The US Center for Disease Control and Prevention reports that up to 90 per cent of all illness and disease is stress-related. When stressed, we're playing out a response from our primal brain, but we do have the option to recalibrate our responses with new reactions and possible outcomes.

Looking at these with a little distance can help us see the repeated cycles that we follow and offer more liberating paths. This isn't a 'good' or 'bad' judgement on our behaviour patterns, but an insight into where we may have got stuck and how to get free.

STRESS FEEDS STRESS

This is chicken-and-egg stuff – the more stressed we are, the more our need for self-care, but the more we act from quick-feed impulses that often don't serve our long-term health. Flip this round and the more we look after ourselves, the less impact stress has on our whole systems and the more likely we are to keep habits that limit these knee-jerk responses.

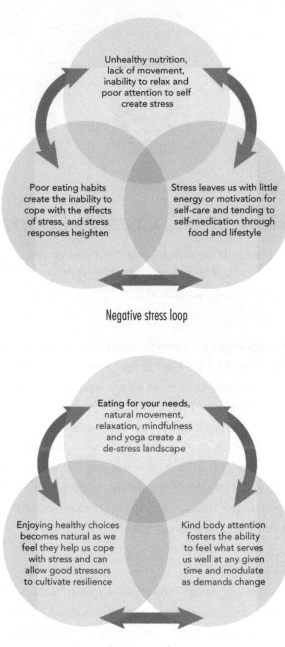

Unhealthy nutrition, lack of movement, inability to relax and poor attention to self create stress

Poor eating habits create the inability to cope with the effects of stress, and stress responses heighten

Stress leaves us with little energy or motivation for self-care and tending to self-medication through food and lifestyle

Negative stress loop

Eating for your needs, natural movement, relaxation, mindfulness and yoga create a de-stress landscape

Enjoying healthy choices becomes natural as we feel they help us cope with stress and can allow good stressors to cultivate resilience

Kind body attention fosters the ability to feel what serves us well at any given time and modulate as demands change

Positive stress loop

The link between your brain, your body and stress

Every time you do anything, from eating a strawberry to checking Twitter, your brain sends messages through nerves to the rest of the body via your spine and out to your organs and limbs. The conscious, muscular part of these actions is your *voluntary nervous system* (VNS). It governs anything you do intentionally, like putting the kettle on, finishing a report or running for the bus.

Another branch of your nervous system is responsible for things that happen without intention, such as blushing or sweating. Called the *autonomic nervous system* (ANS), this also governs your response to stress and has two halves: the *sympathetic nervous system* (SNS) and the *parasympathetic nervous system* (PNS). When someone frightens you, a big tax bill arrives or you're working under pressure, it's your SNS that releases hormones such as adrenaline and cortisol to deliver the energy to handle the problem.

When you're relaxed and calm, sleeping, breathing consciously or listening to soothing music, the PNS is at work rejuvenating your brain and body. So, once the stress has passed, it's the PNS that comes in to reset the chaos and help rebalance your system towards rest and recovery. Calming down helps stimulate digestion, sexual arousal and blood circulation to the skin and extremities. It's why you look and feel better after a deeply restful sleep.

Although much of the ANS action happens automatically, we can consciously make choices to regulate our breathing, diet, lifestyle and mind states to strengthen our PNS and recovery capacity.

The Autonomic Nervous System (ANS)	
Sympathetic nervous system (SNS)	Parasympathetic nervous system (PNS)
Prepares the body for 'fight or flight', emergencies and activity:	Rebuilds the body systems and reverses the changes that the stress response induces:
Release of stress hormones adrenaline and cortisol	Slows heartbeat
Blood redirected from skin to muscles, brain and heart	Lowers blood pressure

(continued)

The Autonomic Nervous System (ANS)	
Sympathetic nervous system (SNS)	**Parasympathetic nervous system (PNS)**
Increases heart rate and blood pressure	Normalizes blood-sugar levels
Rapid breathing	Constricts the pupils
Increases sugar levels in blood and muscles (to fuel 'fight or flight')	Increases blood flow to the skin
Increases sweating	Increases and improves digestion
Tenses muscles	Releases tensed muscles
A sudden rush of strength	Relaxed attitude
Dilated pupils	Improved memory and learning
More sensitive hearing	Tense head and jaw release
Inhibition of non-essential bodily processes – such as digestion, which is slowed down, and sex drive, which is lowered	Allows appropriate immune responses; rest from the inflammation of stress allows fighting of invaders such as bacteria and viruses
Increases production of neurotransmitters: brain chemicals such as serotonin and dopamine that create motivation	Positive outlook as the mind–body can accept that the immediate environment is safe

What stimulates the SNS?	**What stimulates the PNS?**
Rage/anger	Soothing touch
Fear	Meditation and meditative yoga
A looming deadline	Focused breathing
Worry – about family, job, or anything at all	Submersion in water
Exercise that raises heartbeat	Massage
Scary movies	Hypnotherapy
Video games	Acupuncture and acupressure
Situations in which we feel out of control, for example, flying	Essential oils
Phobias	Lying down
Sudden shock or trauma	Sleep
Bright lights and loud noises	Foods that specifically activate it for example, celery
Stimulants – caffeine, nicotine, alcohol, recreational drugs	Slow tempo, 60 bpm music, for example, pieces by Bach or Mozart
Refined sugars	Darkness

Imbalances

Keeping your foot on the gas pedal can cause a state of *sympathetic dominance*, where that 'constant alert' feeling becomes a way of life. But if we live purely in a parasympathetic state we can become listless, demotivated and unresponsive to true stress; this is often seen in those with Chronic Fatigue Syndrome (ME) and burnout, where a tired body enforces 'recovery mode'.

Too much parasympathetic activity from depleted adrenals can damage the very systems it normally takes care of, such as digestion. Finding equilibrium between stimulation and regular recharging rest balances these systems and strengthens your ability to manage stress.

What's your breath telling you?

Here are some common breath-related signs that your nervous system is heightened, and that you need to let the PNS bring you down:

- Hyperventilation – or over-breathing: rapid breath in which you take in more oxygen than the body needs in the face of panic or stress. It can be accompanied by numbness, dizziness, headache and nervous laughter.

- Yawning – this is the body's way of cooling the brain, a signal that you could benefit from a breathing break during cerebral tasks and stressful times.[1]

- Sighing – acts like a reset button for out-of-whack breathing by loosening air sacs that can get tightened by stressed breathing.[2] If you catch yourself sighing often, you may be a breath-holder: your body's way of making up an oxygen deficit.

- Breath-holding – a childhood habit that can stick; we can be unaware we've learned to hold our breath in the face of fear, excitement, even joy, but it creates adrenaline to make us more focused. Notice and breathe deeply – even sigh out with an 'ah' sound – to reset your breath.

- Speaking quickly – Phil Parker, author of *Get the Life You Love, Now,* says 'when you're stressed, if you listen to your voice you'll notice that it will usually be very fast, both if you speak and when you're thinking… just start to slow down your voice and the internal voice of your thoughts, and your breathing will follow'.

Trauma

For some, stress can feel paralysing, and more fear-inducing than the challenge might warrant. Trauma held in the body – from childhood (developmental) or an event (shock) – can activate a more primal part of the brain and nervous system. The 'freeze' response is an alternative to fighting or fleeing and comes from the *primitive vagus system*, a gut reaction to immobilize and 'play dead' that overrides the higher brain functions for language, socialization and even communicating emotional information through the face.

Those whose bodies move into this state can involuntarily feel the need to hide away from people, curl into a foetal ball to feel safe and shut down all responses and connection with others. In his book *In an Unspoken Voice*, trauma specialist Peter Levine states, *'The SNS blocks the social engagement system, but not as completely as the immobilization system.'* Stressful times may periodically force this response upon those with unresolved trauma.

Coming out of this state often involves a 'rebound', with locked-in energy flooding out as irritation, anger and reactive behaviour. If you find yourself caught in these loops, I'd advise seeking specific help through methods like Somatic Experiencing, EMDR (Eye Movement, Desensitization and Reprocessing), EFT (Emotional Freedom Tapping) and/or counselling and hypnotherapy, alongside De-Stress changes, so that trauma can be released 'bottom-up' from your primal brain and processed by your more evolved sympathetic/adrenal systems.

OBSERVING OUR PERSONAL RESPONSE HABITS

Creating awareness in all elements of our lives helps us make sense of our habitual responses. Looking at different ANS expressions then enables us to choose the most appropriate intervention for now and in the broader way we live. Looking at the way our brains respond to a stress or a perceived threat allows us to understand the consequences and how all De-Stress changes – however small – we make can have positive ripple effects.

Stress = mental and physical agitation

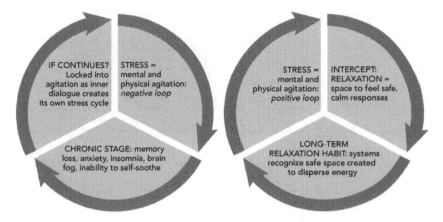

How do I feel?

Reactive and 'buzzy', with the heightened SNS responses described in this chapter and Stressed and Wired on page 53.

- Our brains have a basic resting default setting to continually track our inner (body) and outer environments for potential threats. This baseline vigilance can easily trip over into anxiety if stress is a basic part of our landscape. This world view of 'not safe' can spill over into aggressive speech and action, because our bodies evolved at a time when violence was a part of survival.

- Finding ways to engage the PNS and relaxing feelings of safety that work for you can help relieve this agitation: try warm baths, washing your hands with warm water, self-massage, placing a hand on your heart or rubbing your lips, all of which give instant connection.

- The PNS-related hormone oxytocin is released when we're in love, and by breastfeeding mothers and their babies. It promotes closeness with others. If we don't have enough nurture in our lives, low levels of oxytocin affect our ability to self-soothe. Find physical closeness with others: natural and safe touch with friends, and asking for a hug when you find relaxing your body difficult. Hugging ourselves has the same effect!

Stress = body tension

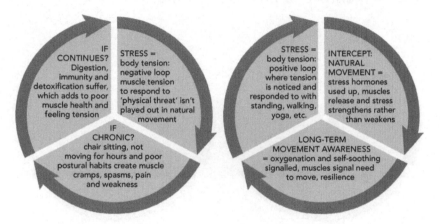

How do I feel?

Tight in the body, face, jaw, head – more on this in chapters 16 and 17.

- Over time, raised levels of cortisol lower the production of the motivating and rewarding neurotransmitter dopamine, leaving us with little joy from activities we once loved, let alone the enthusiasm to go and do them. Adrenaline is made from dopamine, so its continued activation compounds the issue. Yoga and mindful exercise like walking can reduce adrenaline and awaken enthusiasm for movement; vigorous exercise can deploy adrenaline.

- The physical aspects of yoga open your body and help relieve tight muscles and postural shut-down caused by chair-sitting and fear responses. Yoga postures cultivate body connection, strength, fluid response and flexibility. They present a 'good stress' challenge, evoking a positive response from the circulatory system, muscle strength, release and length, hormonal balance and breathing capacity.

Stress = mental constriction

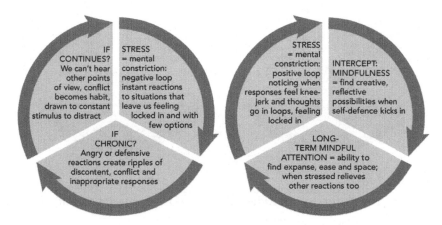

How do I feel?

Locked in, overrun by thoughts, critical and judgemental; see also the mindfulness chapters 13 and 15.

- Stress has us assuming the negative, a crucial survival mechanism in the wild – in the first instance, it was better to think that the shape on the ground was a snake rather than a stick. Today, when stress becomes chronic, that instinct can have us in 'avoid threat' mode rather than 'approach opportunity'. But mindfulness practice has been shown to create an integration between the lower, reptilian brain and the mammalian higher brain, enabling us to retain reason over instinct and the space to lessen knee-jerk reactions to our first thought.

- Stress affects our limbic system, or 'emotional hub', instantaneously, including our ability to integrate thinking and feeling. Within this part of the brain, cortisol stimulates the amygdala, the portion hardwired to focus on the negative and react to it strongly with fear and anger. With less stress, the limbic system can work with the rational brain to blend 'cool' logic working with a 'warm' heart – for example, working out the best strategies for helping others. Meditation has been shown to integrate communication between these mental strengths.

Stress = increased appetite for raised energy needs

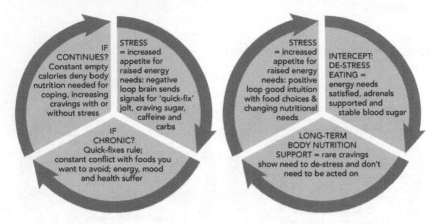

How do I feel?

Driven by the desire to consume, which can be expressed through eating food or in other ways, as explained in Part II.

- There are constant disturbances in our mind–body equilibrium, and our brains are continually sensing what we need in order to restore balance across all systems. Most of the time we don't notice this is happening and it provokes a simple reaction – we feel chilly, so we put on a sweater. But if stress levels are high or our ability to regulate struggles, these needs can enter our consciousness and action is insisted on by the creation of an unpleasant feeling: now we feel painfully cold.

- These heightened senses come with agitation and intense feelings of 'need'. This is the basis of food and other cravings – stress on an overloaded system reads the need to 'refuel' as a screaming desire to self-medicate with chocolate or cake and reset the blood-sugar equilibrium.

- Stress interrupts the dopamine pathways in our brains. This motivation and reward neurotransmitter is released when we come into contact with things we associate with past pleasure. So, feeling comforted when granny gave us a biscuit forged the pathway that says a biscuit could solve things when we are p%&*£d with the world. But we have the choice to feed our brains, instead of trapping them in craving mode. If we create new neural pathways that say, for example, healthy food gives us more energy and vitality, the seeds for new and positive reward cycles are sown.

NOT ALL STRESS IS BAD

As we discussed in chapter 1, stress hormones have a motivating effect on the body, increasing mental acuity, motivation and exuberance, but their supply is finite and their effects depleting. Each stimulus needs a following period of rest and recuperation, so that it can recharge rather than deplete us.[3]

Professor Mark Mattson, from the National Institute on Aging in the US, says that 'the right kind of stress can improve length and quality of life.'[4] Regular exposure to mild stressors, he explains, causes a protective body response that supports its defence systems – including brain, immune, muscle and metabolism function – which might otherwise decline as we age. An example of a mild stressor is weight-bearing exercise, which increases bone density.

This strengthening process, known as *hormesis*, means that by exposing ourselves intermittently to good stress, over time we build mental and physical resilience to protect ourselves against further, bigger challenges.[5,6] Finding balanced and positive ways to deal with stress is more effective than trying to eliminate it from our lives, which can leave us feeling inadequate and disappointed when that proves impossible.

Hearteningly, a German researcher named Gerald Heuther has also suggested that long-term stress may cause people to reject long-held assumptions about themselves or their behaviours and become more open to change.[7] Hans Selye, one of the early pioneers of modern stress theory, called unhealthy, damaging stress *distress* and motivating stress that makes us stronger *eustress*. Here's how to differentiate between this 'good' and 'bad' stress:

Positive stressful challenges

These create excitement, but are short-term enough not to seem relentless and with 'no way out'. Here's what characterizes them:

- They are within our control (or seem to be) – that job interview might be making you sweat and shake, but there's plenty you can do to improve your chances of success, such as researching the company and making sure you sleep well the night before. You can't control the outcome, but you can control your performance.

- They have an end in sight – studying for exams or producing a larger-than-life work project by a certain date are stressful, but they also have an end point.

- They are followed by a period of recuperation – even the most prolific entrepreneurs, athletes and pressured pros need downtime or they risk burnout.

Positive stressors

Being present and able to step away from the need to label things as 'good, bad or neutral' allows us to experience things that build flexible and resilient response mechanisms, including:

- Exercise that challenges your body and is followed by adequate rest.

- Contact with nature where your skin is stimulated by the elements; the odd sting, scratch and irritation may help reset an over-inflammatory system. Dry skin brushing at home can emulate this; see page 111.

- Stretching with breath awareness to learn to stay calm in the face of strong sensations.

- Feeling chilly – the science of *thermogenics* asserts that being cold raises metabolism and modulates immunity. Turning down the heating, taking cold showers and outdoor movement prompt the body to produce 'brown fat', which we burn as fuel, rather than 'white fat', which we store. These things clearly make us more 'hardy' – but do ease in gradually!

- Being hungry between meals – most animals live in a state of perpetual hunger that galvanizes the overriding imperative to find food; eating fewer calories has been shown to increase health and longevity.

- Intellectual challenges in which you feel a sense of control over the situation – and can learn to balance problem-solving with the odd frustration; morning crossword anyone?

Negative stressors

These are situations in which we feel we're 'living on our adrenals'. We can get locked into these patterns and their reactions. Negative stress is:

- Chronic and ongoing – having a mean boss, an unhappy marriage, an isolated or non-existent social life, an unrewarding job or money problems that won't relent.

- Self-judgemental – worrying, ruminating or judging ourselves over mistakes or events; would a friend talk to you like this?

- Out of our control – situations (especially jobs or relationships) in which you feel helpless have been shown to be the most deeply affecting type of stress.

- Excessive physical exertion – keeping the stress response running high and breaking down muscle with no time or energy to rebuild can create an addictive need for the beta endorphin 'high', even when you instinctively know it's wearing you down. See pages 248–49 for how to gauge when exercise is destructive rather than constructive.

ADAPTATION AND RESILIENCE

Hans Selye noted that 'there is [a] type of evolution which takes place in every person during his own lifetime from birth to death: this is the adaptation to the stresses and strains of everyday existence. Through the constant interplay between his mental and bodily reactions, man has it in his power to influence this second type of evolution to a considerable extent.'

Resilience is defined as the ability to cope and adapt in the face of adversity, and to bounce back even when stressors seem overwhelming. Balancing good and bad stress needs constant attention, as it's easy to get caught up in life pressures and to lose sight of when even seemingly selfless giving wears down our ability to engage fully with others.

'Compassion fatigue' is common among those who help others (including nurses and social workers) and resilience research often observes these groups. It's a natural human stress response as a 'safety in numbers' survival tactic, fuelled by the innate urge to protect future generations.

This can be seen more commonly in women – originally the 'gatherers' of the tribe – and interestingly, studies have shown that women are more likely to respond positively to loving-kindness meditation practices like the one on page 189.[8] This isn't to say that men are less capable of compassion, but rather that women may be in more danger of putting others' needs before their own and draining their resources in the process.

Prioritizing self-care – and putting dedicated space in the diary for it – can allow us to be fully present, engaged and caring around others. Listening to music, having a massage, spending time with those who make you feel safe and happy and preparing nourishing food all regulate stress systems; the studies are there, but you don't really need to be told that, do you?

I want to be alone

Knowing what you need in order to recharge is crucial to your personal De-Stress equilibrium. Introverts need to be away from people to recharge and they suffer easily from overstimulation. This isn't the same as shyness – they can enjoy communicating with others, but can feel drained by it and so need to seek regular nights in and quiet time. Extroverts need to seek out healthy contact with people to decompress after stress; feeling alone and isolated can be a source of stress to them.

Opposing and buffering high cortisol

All this talk of the 'dangers' of cortisol begs the question, what brings it down? All actions in the body have an opposing action, without which they would simply continue until the fuel ran out. For cortisol, the 'enough already' signal comes from the 'anti-stress' hormone DHEA (dehydroepiandrosterone), a major marker for age and health.

DHEA's normal effect in a stress-coping person is to bring cortisol back down to baseline, so it's released when a perceived threat has passed. DHEA protects against both immune and autoimmune diseases, including cancer. It's been shown to have significant anti-obesity and anti-diabetic effects, as cortisol raises blood sugar and either spares or enhances the effects of insulin.[9] Prolonged stress eventually leads to low DHEA levels, where people are often observed to have 'lost the joy' in life.

Lifestyle considerations for raising DHEA

Joy, connection, comfortable social contact and anything that our primal systems feel promotes survival of the species have the ability to support adrenal production of DHEA[10,11]

- Blood-sugar balance and adrenal support via stress regulation and the De-Stress Eating guidelines later in the book.

- Be happy – laugh for five minutes, three times a day. Find something that amuses you – a person, a comedy programme on TV or on the radio – and really let go. This is crucial stuff!

- Exercise – build up to 10 minutes of stretching and 45 to 50 minutes of brisk walking on most days of the week.

- Enjoy sex – even fun sexual fantasies are good.

- Get outside for an hour each day, especially if you work inside and/ or are exposed to electronic equipment – computers, printers, cars, planes etc.

- The positive visualization on page 193 has been shown to raise DHEA by encouraging 'thinking with the heart'.

CHAPTER 5

Which Stress Suit Are You Wearing?

'Life is 10% what happens to me and 90% how I react to it.'
<small>JOHN MAXWELL</small>

When stress is chronic and relentless, it begins to compromise our bodily functions with physical and mental symptoms as we struggle to adapt. From catching every cold going to uncomfortable bloating or dog-tiredness, it's likely that you'll see the same old health issues pop up when you're under continuous, intense stress.[1]

The specific nature of how your body expresses symptoms is the Stress Suit you wear.[2] Maybe you've been to the doctor and were told that your symptoms are 'stress-related', but came away not really understanding how or why. Understanding the link between long-term stress and its physiological effects can help you notice personal warning signs and steer away from symptoms.

The seven Stress Suits are:

1. Stressed and Wired

2. Stressed and Tired

3. Stressed and Cold

4. Stressed and Bloated

5. Stressed and Sore

6. Stressed and Demotivated

7. Stressed and Hormonal (women only)

These aren't static states: many people oscillate between two or more. You'll probably identify with more than one Stress Suit as no body system works in isolation, so decide if you want to address the most pressing concern or several at a time. Every change will ripple through.

Follow the De-Stress Eating guidelines in Part II, adding some of the suggestions in this chapter and those at the end of chapter 9. Revisit this chapter from time to time too – noting improvements can remind you that your efforts are getting results.

The checklist of signs and symptoms and the points to prioritize for each Stress Suit (see below) will help you to identify the specific Stress Suit you wear at any given time. They've been compiled using the principles of *functional medicine*, which looks at how imbalances in lifestyle, environment and diet can manifest in the body. This views you as an individual in order to explore underlying causes and offer natural ways to optimize health.[3,4,5]

This advice isn't intended as a substitute for investigation by a qualified nutritional therapist or naturopath (alongside your doctor), who can recommend personal nutritional supplements and tests such as an Adrenal Stress Profile and a saliva test to measure your cortisol and DHEA levels (see last chapter).

At www.charlottewattshealth.com you can access the free ebook De-Stress Supplement Guide, as there's simply not the space in this book to do this subject justice. Generally, a multivitamin and -mineral, vitamin C, omega-3 oil and probiotic supplement are recommended to help everyone cope with the demands of modern life and with extras for the different Stress Suits. Even if you aren't keen on popping pills, this supplement guide has more information about separate nutrients and specific needs if you're vegetarian or vegan.

1. STRESSED AND WIRED

Symptoms and signs:

- being on 'constant alert'
- quick reactions to stressful situations
- little relaxation time or an inability to relax
- feeling the need to constantly 'do'
- long-term life demands and/or emotional stressors
- feeling less 'able to cope'
- mood swings, irritability, thin on patience
- light-, sound- or crowd-sensitive

We all have a little bit of Stressed and Wired in us. Subjecting our nervous systems to constant stimulation from sounds, sights, lights and information from our 24/7 hyper-connectivity, we can be on 'constant alert' without realizing it – with a heightened, wired state feeling 'normal'.[6] But insidiously, it wears out our systems.[7] Adrenal overload can lower levels of the anti-anxiety neurotransmitter gamma-aminobutyric acid (GABA), which is crucial for calm and clarity and often low in those with insomnia, depression and addictions.[8]

If it's not addressed with rest, recovery and nutrition, a Wired Suit can quickly turn to a Tired one (below) and symptoms can take longer to recover from.

If you're a 'doer' or a 'fixer', the list above probably looks familiar. You may be used to pushing through feelings of exhaustion and ignoring your body's signals of tiredness and stress. But this isn't sustainable and having any of the symptoms above shows that you need to start listening to your body and respecting the importance of calming down and occasionally doing nothing.[9] You may struggle with the idea of mindfulness, but this highlights how much you need to let go of the reins sometimes.

Points to prioritize

Slow down – slowly

The first three weeks of De-Stress Eating (see Part II) will help you decrease reliance on stress, sugar and/or stimulants like coffee, alcohol and/or cigarettes for energy that could push you towards Stressed and Tired burnout. Learning to relax and be present is an acquired skill that needs practice, so don't expect suddenly to be able to meditate for hours if you can't sit still for more than two minutes at the moment. A few moments of conscious breathing in the morning or before bed can make all the difference.

Walk

See page 239 on how to prioritize this important activity.

Use evenings to unwind

Look at your evening routines, especially as you're making changes that may take your natural energy a while to kick in. See the advice in chapters 7 and 13 on eating mindfully and calming down before bed.

Snack on celery

Celery's calming effects are a traditional insomnia and anxiety remedy, making it your best snack choice. Research has shown that four stalks of celery a day actively lower blood pressure, as the chemicals apigenin and phthalide expand blood vessels and activate the PNS.[10] It's a good appetite regulator too.

Replace nutrients lost to stress

Zinc, iron, B vitamins, vitamin C and magnesium are commonly lost from the body during the stress response; optimize quality food sources – see chapter 8 – to help feed back the large amounts you utilize to be able to cope with stress.

Magnesium: Our ability to calm and regulate mood via the PNS relies on the mineral magnesium. Deficiency can show up as any symptom relating to nervous system agitation: anxiety, insomnia, headaches, muscle cramps, PMS, depression, fatigue, fibromyalgia, panic attacks, IBS, blood-sugar issues.[11,12,13,14,15] The best sources are green, leafy vegetables, nuts, seeds, fish, carrots, sweet potato, avocado, cauliflower, tahini, parsley, traditionally prepared soy, lentils.

2. STRESSED AND TIRED

Symptoms and signs:

- feeling tired or unrefreshed on waking
- increasing reliance on sugar and/or stimulants for energy
- energy dips
- feeling fuzzy-headed or having 'daytime fog'
- exhaustion in the evening
- feeling cold and sluggish
- sleep disturbances
- fluid retention

Many people living with chronic stress rotate between the Wired and Tired Suits, even within the course of a day. Years of being Wired without rest and recovery can tip over into Tired with low adrenal function (see page 14),[16,17,18] followed by thyroid function upset and metabolic slowing. The result is exhaustion, and weight gain becomes more likely and weight loss harder.[19]

Years of high cortisol can result in crashes that leave you unable to create energy without sugar or stimulants.[20,21] This is a sign that you need to nurture yourself and re-evaluate how you live your life to avoid or come back from burnout.

Points to prioritize

Limit stimulants

You're probably dependent on external energy fixes like stress itself, sugar and/or stimulants like coffee, alcohol or cigarettes. It can seem difficult to give these up when they seem to be the only things keeping you going, but these 'uppers' are wearing you down and depleting nutrients your body and brain rely on to create energy and deal with stress.[22] Cut back gradually as you implement the positive nutritional changes in this book. As you feel better you may want/need external quick fixes less and less often.

Detoxify

Inefficient detoxification, caused and worsened by stagnant metabolic waste products and toxins, could be making you feel sluggish and stopping nutrients getting into cells. See page 110 for more on this.

Rehydrate

Dehydration can make you tired, especially when stressed and getting little water from vegetables and fruit, as well as in drinks (see page 170).

Keep on moving

Increase enjoyment in your life to raise the anti-stress DHEA (see page 49). This hormone relies on regular movement for production; don't think that because you're tired you should never move. Studies show that muscle quickly atrophies without movement and metabolism slows down when it seems that energy production isn't needed. Build up intelligently; see chapter 18.

Have a high-protein breakfast

Try 'Breakfast Outside the Box' on page 135 to provide morning protein, B vitamins, vitamin C and magnesium for energy production and adrenal support.[23]

Eat energy foods

Include the following iron and vitamin B12-rich foods in your diet:

Sources of iron: animal protein – haem (the form from which we can most easily make haemoglobin in blood): red meats, fish, poultry, organ meats, eggs, dairy. Fruit, vegetables, pulses and seeds – non-haem: prunes, dried figs, sesame seeds, tofu, pine nuts, millet, beans (lentils, lima, navy, pinto, black), spinach, watercress. These sources are especially important if you're a vegetarian. Oats, soybeans and fortified cereals and breads also contain non-haem iron, but unless prepared as suggested in the coming chapters, they may inhibit absorption.

Sources of vitamin B12: animal (high) sources: meat, poultry, organ meats, fish, eggs, milk, dairy, seafood. Plant (low) sources of B12 are similar but not as effective – some may even worsen B12 deficiency. Dulse, chlorella, nori, cultured and fermented bean products like tempeh, tofu, miso and also mushrooms show varying amounts.[24]

3. STRESSED AND COLD

Symptoms and signs:

- waking feeling unrefreshed
- less and less energy
- reduction or loss of hearing
- feeling colder than others most of the time
- fluid retention and poor circulation
- hair thinning or loss, especially outer edge of eyebrows
- feeling demotivated and unable to concentrate
- hoarse voice
- hypothyroidism (low thyroid function)

A state of continual 'constant alert' signals the need to conserve energy for potential action. As a survival response to this perceived danger, the adrenal glands tell the thyroid gland to go-slow by down-regulating its output.[25] As the thyroid governs metabolism (the rate at which every body cell burns fuel or calories), lowered function means that weight loss becomes harder and harder.

When the adrenal glands are tired from years of stress, thyroid hormones can struggle to reach body tissues; constant feelings of coldness, poor circulation and fluid retention can result. Since low thyroid function has been shown to lead to heightened feelings of anxiety, this can become a vicious cycle.[26]

If you've been diagnosed with hypothyroidism, regardless of whether you have the symptoms above, taking the advice in this section, alongside other suggestions in the book, may help to improve how you feel. If you're on thyroxine and have had your symptoms relieved by medication, supporting your thyroid naturally is still important. Have your thyroid function regularly tested by your GP, to check your medication levels are still right after making changes to your diet and lifestyle.

Many people may have had a 'normal' result from a doctor's thyroid function test. That's because it's possible to have a thyroid functioning slightly short of the medical classification of hypothyroidism, or because your body isn't utilizing the hormones it does make.[27] If this sounds like you, especially if you have three or more of the symptoms above, chances are you'll benefit from the thyroid-supporting lifestyle changes below.

Points to prioritize

Exercise

This stimulates thyroid hormone secretion and enables your body to pick it up for use. See chapter 19.

Balance blood sugar

Low thyroid function can go hand in hand with insulin resistance and weight piling on, so if you take no other advice from De-Stress Eating, lower your sugar and refined carbohydrate intake and eat quality protein and good fats at each meal to stabilize blood sugar.

Cut back on alcohol or coffee

Try this for a while to see if symptoms improve. Alcohol and coffee interfere with thyroid function, further upsetting blood-sugar balance.[28]

Try targeted yoga

Yoga poses like backbends or inversions (where your head is below your heart) encourage blood flow and delivery of oxygen and nutrients to the thyroid, while encouraging the calming that supports it; see chapter 18.

Avoid uncooked 'goitrogenic' foods

When eaten raw, cabbage, Brussels sprouts, broccoli, cauliflower, turnips, mustard greens, collards and kale interfere with thyroid function and can enlarge it.[29] However, they're extremely beneficial to the thyroid when cooked, as they support liver function – and thyroid hormones are activated in the liver.[30] Soy is also goitrogenic.

Hot up

Low thyroid function reduces the amount of heat produced as energy in cells; the thermogenic measures on page 46 force the body to make its own heat. Go for a brisk walk in the cold, even when you don't feel like it!

Add tyrosine

The amino acid (protein building block) tyrosine is needed to make the thyroid hormone thyroxine with the mineral iodine (see food sources below), and relies on food sources from protein and leafy greens such as kale, collards and spinach. Tyrosine is also used to make adrenaline and noradrenaline (released in response to stress), leaving less available for the thyroid when these are raised.

Thyroid-supporting nutrients

These include iron, zinc, copper and selenium[31,32], which can be depleted through a non-organic, grain-rich or some long-term vegetarian diets. Replacing these with the vegetable and protein sources recommended in De-Stress Eating (and a multivitamin and mineral supplement) helps these minerals to work with iodine to create and utilize thyroxine.

Sources of iodine: high amounts are found in mackerel, cod, shellfish and lobster. Some seaweeds, such as kelp or kombu, are rich forms of iodine (nori, dulse and arame usually test low). Buy organic as they absorb toxic metals. Moderate amounts are found in butter, eggs, goat's cheese and yoghurt. Note: even in iodized salt, the iodine can quickly evaporate; the good-quality sea salt recommended in the book isn't iodized.

4. STRESSED AND BLOATED

Symptoms and signs:

- bloating and/or gas after eating
- digestive or Irritable Bowel Syndrome (IBS)-type symptoms worsen when stressed
- food sensitivities
- constipation and/or diarrhoea – lack of daily 'full and satisfying evacuation'
- headaches
- poor digestion of fats and/or greasy or pale-coloured stools
- frequent or long-term use of steroid medications, anti-inflammatories and/or antibiotics
- diet high in sugar, refined carbohydrates and/or grains

Gut health influences all other body systems, from immunity to our ability to deal with stress.[33] The inflammation, poor detoxification and hormone imbalance that can result from an unhealthy digestive environment are stressors in themselves.[34] That environment relies on the presence of around 3kg (7lb) of beneficial or 'probiotic' bacteria – heavier than all of your skin cells. These *good* bacteria are quickly lowered by stress, sugar, alcohol, antibiotics and steroid medications[35,36], leading to food intolerances, digestive issues and weight gain.

During stress, low levels of beneficial gut bacteria can prompt inflammation in those susceptible[37]; a growing body of evidence shows links between inadequate levels and conditions such as asthma, eczema and arthritis.

The stress response immediately diverts energy, oxygen and nutrients away from the gut and skin towards the brain and muscle. Digestion is activated by the calming vagus nerve, which runs directly from brain to gut, ordering an immediate muscular contraction of digestive muscles. While digestion initially slows when stress hits, ongoing and chronic stress can cause spasm or constriction of gut muscles or uncomfortable cycles of diarrhoea and constipation as the gut struggles for balance.[38]

Points to prioritize

Pay attention to how you eat

More mindful, calm eating is a De-Stress cornerstone (see page 93). Thoroughly chewed food has the best chance of complete digestion and less chance of causing food intolerances. It also helps the brain register 'full' signals before you've overeaten.[39]

Reduce stimulants

Refined sugars, stress, alcohol and excess caffeine compromise probiotic bacteria levels, which can lead to gas production, poor immunity and overgrowths of yeasts such as *Candida albicans*. Always wait an hour after eating heavy protein before having fruit, or gut fermentation can develop, causing gas. Stick to berries for least reaction.

Increase prebiotics

These are foods that feed your probiotic gut bacteria and have been shown to help your gut cope with stress[40] and lead to weight loss through appetite control.[41] You'll get loads by increasing your vegetable intake, but the highest levels of the prebiotic inulin are found in Jerusalem artichokes, chicory, bananas, garlic, onions, leeks, kiwi fruit and dandelion leaves (for weeding gardeners out there). Prebiotics have also been shown to help reduce the negative effects of a diet previously too low in omega-3 oils – which may affect the gut's ability to heal itself.

Use herbs and spices

Ginger, mint, turmeric and other herb leaves and spices contain volatile oils that give them their pungent smell and have a calmative effect on the gut. Add herbs liberally to salads and make fresh herb and spice teas rather than sugary soft drinks to lower your sugar intake. Parsley aids fluid retention and bloating as it helps rid the body of excess water, uric acid, salt and toxins by virtue of the plant chemicals it contains called *apiol* and *myristicin*.

Watch your intake of gluten

Found mostly in wheat, but also in spelt, kamut, rye and barley, and used in many processed foods and additives (such as dextrin and malt), gluten can cause gut problems. Bran has been shown to worsen IBS.[42] A severe gluten intolerance can lead to coeliac disease, where the gut lining is damaged, but gluten has also been linked to IBS and inflammatory conditions, including skin problems.[43,44,45]

Eat fewer lectins

Lectins are sugar-binding proteins (like gluten, above) found in whole grains, beans, dairy and potatoes, as well as nightshade vegetables and peanuts. They are often involved in food allergies and sensitivities and can contribute to low energy and weight gain by disabling cells in the gastrointestinal tract, keeping them from repairing and rebuilding.[46]

Some people tolerate lectins while others may find they put a strain on their digestion, particularly if they tend to gas and bloating. In the six-week De-Stress Eating plan in Part II, you'll be replacing lectin-rich foods with more vegetables and exploring how that makes you feel.

Get tested

Dairy, eggs, fish and grains are common foods that cause food intolerance, which is a delayed immune response – different from an immediate, obvious allergy. Food intolerances can change, especially as stress lowers and the gut heals. But you might want to consider an IgG blood test (which tests for the antibody produced in food intolerance) if symptoms persist, as they are almost impossible to self-diagnose. See www.charlottewattshealth.com for more details.

5. STRESSED AND SORE

Symptoms and signs:

- inflammatory conditions such as hay fever, asthma, eczema, arthritis or psoriasis
- frequent infections, including ear, nose and throat
- Irritable Bowel Syndrome and other digestive conditions
- bloating, fluid retention and sudden weight fluctuations
- frequent or long-term use of steroid medications, anti-inflammatories and/or antibiotics

- diet high in sugar, refined carbohydrates and/or grains
- degenerative conditions such as osteoporosis, heart disease, joint problems
- autoimmune conditions such as MS, diabetes, lupus

Low-level inflammation is at the root of many aspects of poor health, weight gain and chronic disease.[47,48] Even if you don't see obvious external inflammation, stress and poor dietary habits can set off an inflammatory cascade in tissues and blood vessels that contributes to symptoms.[49,50,51,52]

Our gut lining is home to the antibody secretory-IgA, one of our few anti-inflammatory mechanisms, which relies on healthy levels of gut bacteria or can signal overreaction by the immune system, setting off inflammation and food sensitivities and intolerances.[53] See the Stressed and Bloated section above and a nutritional therapist can use a stool test to investigate and support the health of your gut environment.

If you're in inflammatory mode, your energy may be sapped by your immune system being on overdrive. This can cause 'cytokine sickness', where the constant signalling of the body's immune messengers in response to inflammation can lead to a feeling of being generally unwell, in the form of low-level flu symptoms, low mood and skin conditions that won't shift.[54,55,56,57]

Eating quickly, not fully chewing food and/or eating when stressed can mean food enters the gut only partially broken down. There it sits around, contributing to an imbalance of bacteria, gas-production, bloating, constipation, food sensitivities and IBS. This is a recipe for toxicity and inflammation.

Points to prioritize

Reduce sugar

This will reduce the production of inflammatory AGEs (advanced glycation end-products), created in response to sugar and stress. These can contribute to the ageing of every cell in the body (including the skin) by 'cross-linking' or lost movement within cells.[58] Sugar also disrupts white blood cell production, reducing your ability to fight infection.

Choose antioxidants

Our ancestors ate high levels of antioxidants.[59] These are naturally occurring chemicals that counteract the harmful 'oxidizing' effects of stress, pollution, sunlight, eating burned (like barbecued) and fried foods and everyday chemicals. We need more antioxidants when exercising too, for recovery and preventing the inflammation that can lead to injury.

De-Stress Eating is chock-full of foods that provide antioxidant nutrients such as vitamin C, vitamin E, beta-carotene, glutathione, selenium and zinc, as well as specific bioflavonoids and polyphenols in spices, black tea, green tea and garlic alongside antioxidant-rich treats like red wine and dark chocolate.

Hydrate

Dehydration can signal the production of inflammation signalling histamine (see page 170).

Watch the lectins

See Stressed and Bloated, above. Those susceptible to inflammation can react to the specific lectins in grains, beans and the nightshade vegetable family (which includes tomatoes, potatoes, red peppers and aubergines).[60,61] These lectins are lessened when cooked but try avoiding or reducing these foods if you have signs of inflammation, especially joint pain.[62]

Get your omega-3 oils

Low omega-3 and high omega-6 can lead to inflammation. Those with conditions such as eczema, asthma, dermatitis, hay fever, migraines and arthritis may have difficulty converting plant sources of omega-3 and omega-6 into the anti-inflammatory, healing prostaglandins needed to get their full benefits; stress compounds this. See omega-3 food sources on page 100.[63,64]

6. STRESSED AND DEMOTIVATED

Symptoms and signs:

- poor motivation and get-up-and-go
- tendency to depression

- feeling less positive than before
- using sugar and refined carbs for comfort
- late-night binges or overeating sessions
- sleeping issues
- wanting to withdraw from the world
- Seasonal Affective Disorder (SAD)

The brain is energy-rich, demanding around 25–70 per cent of our fuel intake (stress takes it up to the higher end of that). Stress also creates cravings for quick fixes as the brain tries to self-medicate to compensate for an inconsistent fuel supply from blood-sugar imbalance,[65] provoking more cravings, mood swings and a vicious cycle of 'using' sugar and stimulants to keep our minds going.

This scenario limits nutrients available to the brain, including magnesium, zinc, iron, B vitamins and vitamin C. These are required to create neurotransmitters such as serotonin and dopamine – or 'happy chemicals' – which are vital for focus, alertness and mood stability. Those who tend towards low levels of these neurotransmitters often get more of a kick from stimulating or numbing substances such as alcohol, junk food, recreational drugs and addictive medication like benzodiazepines (the highly addictive Valium family).

These habits, alongside stress, give us a sudden rise in the feel-good brain chemicals GABA, dopamine and serotonin, but cause crashes later, leading to cycles of dependence and an increasing reliance on them in order to 'feel normal'.[66] These craving cycles also cause weight gain,[67] which can lower self-esteem and feed into habits of bingeing and/or overeating.[68]

This is your biochemistry at work.[69] It's inaccurate to blame yourself or your lack of willpower. Excess weight has been shown to contribute to depression,[70] so positive steps to get slim and stay calm can help on many levels. Low or imbalanced neurotransmitters upset appetite regulation, intuitive eating and feelings of fullness or satisfaction – see more about cravings in chapter 7.[71]

Points to prioritize

Eat protein with each meal

Ensuring consistent energy to the brain is the cornerstone of good mental health. Eating protein with every meal ensures neurotransmitter production to be able to create and maintain positive mood, feelings of motivation and a desire to socialize.

Address sugar intake

Sugar addiction cycles can be aggressive in those who tend to have low serotonin levels. Serotonin is crucial to our sleep and mood cycles, so inadequate levels trigger a sugar-craving survival mechanism for a quick fix; this raises insulin needed to increase serotonin in the brain. De-Stress Eating focuses on relieving these cycles.

Mind your gut

Explore Stressed and Bloated advice above. Even if you don't have those symptoms, there's a strong gut-brain connection. Evidence shows that replenishing probiotic gut bacteria also helps alleviate mild depression, as inflammatory processes that start in the gut produce immune messengers that can have depressive effects on the brain.[72]

Increase your omega-3s

DHA, an omega-3 fatty acid found in fish oil (e.g. salmon and mackerel), is the most abundant fat in the brain and is known to be essential for serotonin receptors and dopamine levels. Low dopamine and serotonin are linked to depression and other mental health issues.[73]

Find natural highs

Natural opioids or 'beta-endorphins' are produced in response to laughing, music, socializing, hugs and sex, a fabulous reward system for keeping the species going. Unfortunately sugar causes a surge of these, too, so it can be even more difficult to give that up when we aren't creating our own beta-endorphins.

Get out and get moving

See page 244 for the benefits of outdoor exercise. Cortisol affects our ability to uptake vitamin D3[74] which is needed for mood regulation and associated with Seasonal Affective Disorder (SAD) or 'winter blues' when we don't get enough sunlight on the skin.

Vitamin D3 sources: the best source is sunlight, see page 244 for guidelines. High amounts found in mackerel, salmon, trout, herring; moderate amounts in eggs. Note: cow's milk and other dairy foods are fortified with D3 in the USA but not the UK.

7. STRESSED AND HORMONAL – FOR WOMEN ONLY

Symptoms and signs:

- PMS or a history of menstrual problems

- periods becoming heavier, more painful, less regular

- female hormone issues, for example, fibroids, endometriosis, Polycystic Ovary Syndrome (PCOS)

- premenstrual or ovulation sugar cravings

- menopausal symptoms

- fertility issues

- long-term use of oral, IUD or injected hormonal contraception

- hormonal phases of irritability, crying and/or negative thoughts

If your sex hormones are unbalanced, chances are you also scored highly for some of the preceding Suits. That's because your adrenal glands and thyroid directly affect the balance of oestrogen and progesterone in your body, and when they become unbalanced through stress, heavy, painful periods and other hormonal symptoms may result.[75,76] This is because cortisol and other stress hormones depend on progesterone for their production, which can skew the delicate balance your hormonal system needs to function well. It can also lead to weight gain in 'female areas' like the bottom, hips and thighs.

Stress can also raise male 'androgenic' hormones in women, leading to male-shaped weight around the middle, menstrual and menopausal problems and Polycystic Ovary Syndrome (PCOS). The De-Stress Effect optimizes liver function, digestion and blood-sugar balance, which consequently helps hormonal regulation.[77]

Points to prioritize

Liver support

Optimizing detoxification increases your ability to break down and release used hormones from the body (see page 110 for more information).

Digestive system support

Looking after your digestion also supports the liver, encouraging elimination of toxins and excess hormones via the bowel. It also helps address any constipation that could be causing used hormones and toxins to be reabsorbed into the body. Try the Bircher muesli medley on page 136 and add in soaked linseeds for hormone-balancing lignans.[78]

Eat some soy (but don't overdo it)

You might be confused about the conflicting health messages regarding soy for female hormone issues and menopausal health. Traditional fermented forms – such as soy sauce, tamari (gluten-free soy sauce), miso, tempeh and natto – have long been associated with female health.[79] But traditionally, the Chinese and Japanese only ate soy once they had learned to ferment it – to reduce the phytic acid and lectins – and tofu and miso are traditionally eaten in small amounts as an accompaniment to meals containing meat or fish.

Soy can interfere with zinc absorption and affect our ability to balance all hormones – sexual, adrenal, thyroid and blood-sugar balance – as well as affecting tissue-healing and fertility.[80] Practically speaking, eating traditional soy foods several times weekly can help female hormone-balance regulation, but avoid soy in other processed forms like soy milk and soy protein isolate and textured vegetable protein (TVP). These are used to make 'fake' meat products and tend to be high in toxins and can upset hormone-balancing abilities.

Watch the alcohol

Alcohol can raise circulating oestrogen and may worsen PMS and heighten breast cancer risk, especially if you take it in drip-feed amounts and find that nightly glass often turns into half a bottle – see page 175.[81]

Choose organic meat, eggs and dairy

It's more expensive but worth it, and if you can only make one organic choice make it this. Non-organic meat, eggs and dairy are higher in the growth and steroid hormones that disrupt our hormone balance.[82,83]

PART II

De-Stress Eating Every Day

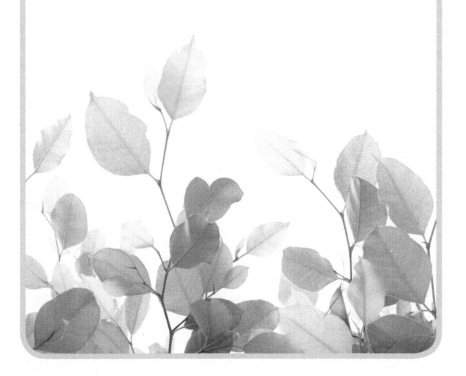

CHAPTER 6

De-Stress Eating Principles

*'Nothing in biology makes sense
except in light of evolution.'*
THEODOSIUS DOBZHANSKY

For many of us, confused appetites, tastes and cravings add up to a stressful relationship with food, the very thing that should be nourishing us. We live in a world with so much choice, it has our brain racing just to decide what to put in our mouth next, and it constantly prompts us to want more. As knee-jerk (mindless, rather than mindful) reactions often result in less nutritious food choices, stress can keep us away from the very foods that help us cope with its effects.

De-Stress Eating is designed to draw you round a complete circle of sustenance. If you're providing your body with the resources it needs in order to cope, you'll be less prey to the impulses that keep you in roller-coaster mode and at the mercy of cravings. This isn't about 'right or wrong' food choices, but about discovering what suits you; it's about truly finding what makes you feel good, so you'll want to keep it up – without rigidity or stress.

Forging a closer relationship with the food you eat can also cultivate the sensitization to truly taste and appreciate the subtleties of healthy, real and wholesome food, creating a feedback loop of contentment rather than self-criticism around your food choices.

HUNTER-GATHERERS AND US

De-Stress Eating is derived from a hunter-gatherer diet (often referred to as a Paleo or Stone Age diet) with the following considerations:

- The recognition that we're no longer living as our ancestors did and that the foods available and the lives we lead are similar in few ways.

- Making the best updates/revisions possible to the Paleo diet while honouring these ancient biorhythms, but without adding the neurosis of 'perfection' to our list of stresses.

- Our bodies evolved to expect different amounts of food on different days and at different times, depending on energy needs and food availability. That's the only 'one size fits all' evidence available to us about what suits the human body.[1,2]

- Considering ways of eating foods relatively new to the human body – like grains and beans – by preparing them in traditional ways and eating them in the amounts that are best tolerated: a more *flexi-Paleo* attitude.

It isn't possible to know how much your own body's genetic history was adapted to more modern foods, but do look to your traditional cultural diet if you know it. Everyone is different and we can see that different people respond in varied ways to the same diets.

According to the Paleo diet's pioneers, such as Boyd Eaton and Dr Loren Cordain, we're 'Stone Agers living in a Space Age'. Although our bodies have slowly adapted in some ways to our modern lives and environments over the last 12,000 years, our basic physiology is still set to eat, move and live in the way that our early ancestors did.[3] The field of genetics is now understanding that our diet and lifestyle choices have an actual impact on the way our genes express throughout our lives, making us more susceptible to weight gain and disease.[4] By choosing to eat, live, move and relax in a way that's more in keeping with our ancestors' lifestyle, we can build a better resistance to modern life and the stress that comes with it.[5]

Our bodies desire food, as that provided motivation for the huge amount of time and energy our ancestors needed to hunt or gather it. Our physiology and biochemistry were established at a time when food was scarce and certainly not as easy to obtain as it is for us today. Our hunter-gatherer ancestors living in the Stone Age – or Paleolithic era (pre-10,000BCE) – would have worked extremely hard for each and every calorie they ate, and everything would have been seasonal, unprocessed and naturally nutrient-dense.

The amount of food they took in would have varied day to day, depending on food sources and energy expenditure, which is estimated to have been three to five times that of the average twenty-first-century Westerner.[6] That's why sticking with the same amount and type of food for weeks or months can mean weight loss efforts become difficult and weight plateaus, especially with stress in the equation[7]; we are used to having to adapt.

Our ancestors' diet would have been packed with levels of vitamins, minerals, antioxidants, soluble fibre and omega-3 oils that we struggle to attain in ours.[8] We know this because nutritional scientists are now looking beyond the effects of what we're eating today to learn from evolutionary biology, anthropology, archaeology and geography and increase our understanding of how our ancestors lived, ate and moved.

This research has shown that our ancestors had lowered levels of obesity, heart disease, cholesterol, depression, cancer, osteoporosis and inflammatory conditions such as acne. Their body composition and fitness were also superior, with less body fat.[9,10,11,12,13]

Some scientists now believe the Western 'diseases of civilization', or 'mismatch diseases'[14], have their roots in inflammatory processes and the poor blood-sugar control that comes as a result of our modern diet. This tends to exacerbate, rather than strengthen, our reactions to the perpetual stress we're under as we struggle to control our blood sugar; our survival mechanisms (such as laying down fat for lean times) can work against instead of for us.

The advent of farming as a way of life took hold on a large scale around 10,000 years ago. In his book *The Story of the Human Body*, Daniel Lieberman, Harvard professor of evolutionary biology, says: 'Farming may have led to civilization and other types of "progress", but… most of the mismatch diseases from which we currently suffer stem from the transition from hunting and gathering to farming.'

This lifestyle shift changed our diet and introduced grains, beans, potatoes, dairy and domesticated meats as staples. Eventually, following the Industrial Revolution of the eighteenth and nineteenth centuries, refined sugar, fat and processed food intake rose rapidly. In evolutionary terms, 10,000 years isn't long at all. This is the key reason our bodies aren't thriving on our modern diet or living habits – true genetic adaptation takes *millions* of years.

STRESS AND THE MODERN DIET

There are several reasons why the composition of our modern diet doesn't suit our stressful lives:

- Low-quality fats from highly domesticated and processed meats, dairy, refined vegetable oils and processed foods provide more saturated fats and fewer anti-inflammatory omega-3 oils than wild meat, game, fish, nuts and eggs.

- Lower protein levels from these unhealthy fat sources promote poor body composition and a higher fat-to-muscle ratio, exacerbated by constant stress that also leads to weight gain and decreased muscle.

- Too many carbohydrates from grains, beans, potatoes and refined sugars, and too few from vegetables, fruit and nuts, can lead to more inflammation and add to the heightened insulin response that leads to the fat storage caused by raised stress hormones.

- Too few nutrients from poor-quality and imbalanced macronutrients (carbohydrates, fats and proteins) lead to lower levels of vitamins, minerals, antioxidants and omega-3 oils, which are also used up in larger amounts during times of stress.

- The high sodium-to-potassium mineral levels in modern foods – from fewer vegetables and fruit – lead to acidity in the body. This is worsened by the poor breathing patterns that happen involuntarily when we're stressed. An acidic system leads to cravings, mood swings, weight gain and bone loss.

- High-sugar, low-soluble fibre carbohydrates, such as grains and processed foods – instead of vegetables, fruit and nuts – heighten the blood-sugar imbalances, energy and mood 'highs and lows' caused by stress hormones.

The traditional people of the Greek island of Crete (pre-1960) – who ate the *real* healthy Mediterranean diet – obtained 35–40 per cent of their calories from fat.[15] They consumed high levels of monounsaturated fats (from olive oil, olives, avocados and nuts), which have been shown to reduce levels of harmful fats circulating in the blood when they replace high carbohydrates. The result was a low incidence of heart disease and obesity.

Other fats, from fish, eggs, nuts and some meat, gave a balanced ratio of higher omega-3 fatty acids than omega-6 and healthy forms of saturated fat. Grains came mainly in the form of sourdough bread, with a little weekly pasta, and less milk but more cheese. They ate meat, eggs and dairy from animals in natural pasture rather than grain-fed, with naturally higher omega-3 oils.

In the Greek countryside, chickens wandered on farms, eating grass, insects, worms and dried figs, all good sources of omega-3 fatty acids and very different to the diet of a sedentary, grain-fed battery farm chicken. Vegetables and fruits were from wild plants, providing high-soluble fibre and anti-inflammatory nutrients such as selenium, glutathione and vitamins E and C.

If we can opt for similar ways of eating as a default, taking our hardware back to 'factory setting', we can explore what suits us, what we can handle when stress hits and what triggers stress-related food cravings.

The modern hunter-gatherer vegetarian

Where does this leave the vegetarian or vegan, who may be concerned about where all this talk of 'man as predator' is going? I assure you there will be no preaching about including foods you don't want to eat – that would be a sure source of stress. You need to feel in balance with anything you put in your body, and mindfulness will help these intuitive decisions. Vegetarians and vegans should pay extra attention to diet and lifestyle measures, as well as the supplement suggestions at www.charlottewattshealth.com, to fully feel The De-Stress Effect.

Although our ancestors were not vegetarian, we can modify the Paleo diet with intelligence to support such ethical choices. Some vegetarians question whether they may need some meat after periods of prolonged or intense stress. When energy, mood and focus wane, the body can crave foods to make up the deficit, and the nutrients used up quickly by the stress response are found in lower amounts in a plant-based diet. If your choice is not to eat meat or fish, ethically sourced eggs are a good alternative.

THE BUILDING BLOCKS: MACRO- AND MICRONUTRIENTS

The main bulk of our food comes from macronutrients, those we need in larger amounts: carbohydrates, proteins and fats. We can create energy from all three, but carbohydrates predominantly. Fats and proteins are also used for the continual growth of skin, bone, muscles, organs and all body cells.

Our ancestors' diet was higher in brain-building proteins and fats; the level of plant foods eaten by chimps and gorillas can lead to gas, bloating and inflammation in humans. Plus we no longer have the teeth size or jaw strength for the chewing this requires – a chimpanzee will spend nearly half its waking time masticating.

Anthropological studies have noted that our larger brains and shorter digestive tracts distinguish us from other primates. This happened as a result of moving to hunting and incorporating more nutrient-dense meat in our diets. As Dan Lieberman says, *'by incorporating meat in the diet and relying more on food processing (chopping, cooking) early Homo sapiens was able to spend much less energy digesting its food and could thus devote more energy towards growing a larger brain.'*[16]

The modern diet industry has fixated on ratios of fats-to-proteins-to-carbs for decades. From the simplistic view that as fats contain more calories than carbohydrates they must cause weight gain grew the high-carbohydrate/low-fat diets of the 1980s and 1990s.[17] Our lean ancestors didn't eat this way and numerous studies have now linked this high-carbohydrate diet with weight gain, as it increases fat storage.[18] Fat – unlike carbs – increases the satisfaction we feel after a meal.[19]

There's also a growing realization that the *micronutrients* you eat – the vitamins, minerals, omega oils, amino acids and others needed in only small amounts – have a significant effect on your metabolism, mood, appetite and weight. Metabolism and weight management aren't as simple as calories burned equals energy expended.[20]

Our body's hormone levels and energy-burning rates are always changing, along with our appetite needs. Healthy adrenal glands, thyroid, brain, pancreas and liver are essential to the way your body adapts to daily demands, with stress both tiring them and depleting the amount of micronutrients they can draw upon. Nor are these micronutrients easily acquired from a high-carbohydrate, low-fat diet.

Protein for satisfaction and thermogenesis

The nutritional CV of quality protein is impressive. This muscle-building, energy-giving macronutrient aids loss of stored fat, satisfies appetite and creates fat-burning heat, or *thermogenesis*, while promoting muscle-building.[21,22,23] Our ancestors would have eaten more and better-quality sources of protein than we do, obtaining it from both dense, wild animal sources including meat, fish, organ meats, shellfish, eggs and insects, and from many more alkalizing plant sources.

Scientists have studied tribes of people on contemporary versions of hunter-gatherer diets and found they have not only improved long-term weight loss but also lowered risk of cardiovascular disease and Type 2 diabetes.[24,25,26,27] Current recommendations of 15 per cent calorie intake from protein are at odds with our ancestors' intake of an estimated 15–30 per cent.[28]

Protein and fat help us handle carbs

The presence of slower-to-digest fat and protein in a meal means the slower release of carbohydrates, which results in better blood-sugar balance.[29] When you're under stress, this is essential. The more carbohydrates in a meal, the more insulin is needed to get the sugar – as glucose – from the broken-down carbohydrates into your bloodstream and then your cells for energy. As insulin rises, blood glucose levels drop.

A high-carbohydrate meal can result in an insulin surge, which means this drop happens suddenly. This sudden low blood glucose, or *reactive hypoglycaemia*, signals a need to find more food. Survival mechanisms then override rational thought, forcing the most direct route to a quick blood-glucose rise: sugar or stimulants like caffeine, alcohol or cigarettes.[30,31] This keeps us locked in the stress response and needing to eat between meals.

Too much insulin = too much fat

After a sugar surge, we can use some of the glucose that floods the bloodstream as energy and store some as glycogen in the muscles and liver, but any excess beyond that is converted to fat. High insulin levels keep us in fat-storing mode – and if we also move our bodies too little we have a recipe for long-term weight gain. Moderating your insulin response by eating little sugar and fewer refined carbohydrates means your body will use up stored fat more efficiently.

The highs and lows of a high-sugar and refined carbohydrate and/or grain diet mean your body and brain receive inconsistent glucose energy supplies. This can quickly affect mood and feed into sugar-addiction cycles that cause cravings, anxiety, insomnia and weight gain. Long term, this raised insulin production can eventually lead to saturated insulin receptor sites, which can no longer pick up the insulin hormone, a state called 'Insulin Resistance' or 'Metabolic Syndrome'. This is on the rise and is linked to diabetes, weight gain around the waist and heart health problems.

As insulin fails to move sugars out of the bloodstream they must be converted to fat, so likelihood of the above conditions increases. This is exacerbated by stress hormones but alleviated by exercise, and by reducing your intake of high-insulin-response foods such as grains, dairy and sugars.[32] Many of the micronutrients in vegetables, fruits, lean meat, nuts and spices have properties that help insulin sensitivity and are an important part of De-Stress Eating, especially if we want the occasional sugary treat.

Clarity on carbohydrates

Our hunter-gatherer ancestors ate about 65 per cent plant foods. These carbohydrate sources would have consisted of vegetables, fruit, nuts, seeds and edible raw roots, which I advise you to increase as your main carbohydrate sources. Many people think that carbohydrates come only from what are really starchy carbs (grains, beans and potatoes), but all plant foods provide carbohydrates, with lactose in dairy the only animal sugar source.

The starches in grains, cereals, beans, peas, corn and roots that need to be cooked (potatoes, tapioca, sweet potatoes, parsnips, yams) aren't believed to have been introduced into the human diet in any significant quantities until farming, harvesting and cooking became widespread (although humans have cooked foods for around 790,000 years).[33] The plants we eat now are starchier, domesticated versions of those that grow wild. Refined sugars, processed foods and desserts weren't a common feature until the Middle Ages.

Vegetables: leaves, stalks and edible roots

There are many properties in vegetables that help enhance the digestibility and absorption of the nutrients in grains and cereals. But most people eat too many grains and too few vegetables, which can lead to digestive problems and nutrient deficiencies.

Eating many more vegetables with smaller amounts of grains and beans (or none at all) reduces the amount of insulin produced and makes the carbohydrates in the plant sources less likely to lead to fat storage and diabetes.[34] Soluble fibre in vegetables, nuts and fruit has recently been associated with a loss of belly fat.[35]

The trouble with grains/cereals and beans/legumes

Grains (wheat, rye, rice, oats, etc.) and beans (soy, pinto, chickpea, green peas, etc.) are relatively new to the human diet; they were only eaten in sparse amounts before our ancestors stopped their nomadic hunter-gatherer lifestyles to stay in one place and cultivate them. We've processed these 'novel foods' more and more as we've moved towards the modern Western diet, to the point where they now dominate it, especially in the form of fast food.

Lectins

These chemicals found in grains and beans cause the immune systems of susceptible people to respond with inflammation and can contribute to weight gain and digestion problems.[36] Lectins have been widely associated with *leptin* resistance – leptin is a hormone that acts as a signal to the brain to inhibit food intake and register fullness. As lectins have also been shown to bind to leptin, they can contribute to loss of appetite control, obesity and diabetes.[37]

Phytic acid

This is a substance which studies have shown inhibits the body's absorption of minerals such as calcium, iron, zinc and magnesium; it also affects its ability to digest protein fully.[38,39,40] When grains and beans comprise more than 50 per cent of our diet, mineral deficiencies can result in rickets, tooth decay and osteoporosis.[41,42,43] This can be worse for those with lower levels of beneficial, probiotic gut bacteria.[44]

While refined grain products such as white rice, pasta and bread are lower in phytic acid and lectins, they create an insulin surge and offer little nutritional value, so undoubtedly add to weight and health issues. If you choose to eat grains for energy purposes, switch from refined ones to small amounts of whole grains.

Traditional farming cultures always neutralized these anti-nutrients by soaking, sprouting, fermenting or naturally leavening beans and grains.[45] This meant that any breads, porridges, stews, grain or bean flours were also cooked slowly or with natural acidifiers (see chapter 10). You'll explore what level is right for you in the six-week De-Stress Eating plan, but even simply moving your vegetable-to-grain/bean ratio towards more vegetables has positive implications for increased detoxification, more favourable alkalinity in your blood, healthier mineral levels and more soluble fibre for a healthier gut.

Moving away from low fat

The weight-loss wars of the last few decades have focused on high-carb/low-fat vs high-protein/low-fat.[46] But the often recommended low-fat diet – high in vegetables, fruit and whole grains – has shown only a small heart disease risk reduction.[47] Recommendations for the blanket reduction of all saturated fat were born of poorly reported evidence that it leads to heart disease and weight gain, when those who restrict it are shown to weigh more.[48,49,50]

This focus on calorie reduction has driven general weight-loss and health guidelines to recommend that we get 30 per cent or less of our calorie intake from fats. But our hunter-gatherer ancestors derived between 28 and 58 per cent of their energy from them.[51,52]

Fat is a quality, not a quantity, issue. We are made of fats, especially our fat-rich brains, and they need to be replenished. But high fat intake from sources such as sedentary, grain-fed animals, and damaged 'trans' fats from fried and processed foods, poses risks of increased cancer, liver and heart disease, especially in a diet also high in sugar. This combination has shown a rise in liver disease in developed countries, even in children.[53] The right fats, on the other hand, are essential to mood, weight stabilization, appetite satisfaction and overall health.

Fat facts

Fats are energy-rich and for our ancestors they would have represented more pay-off for energy spent finding them; their dense, micronutrient-rich sources would have kept 'stoking the fire' in terms of heat production and metabolism. Our ancestors would have eaten leaner meats from wild animals with quality muscle and naturally lower fat levels with much higher omega-3 fatty acid levels.[54]

Omega-3 oils contain the essential fatty acids DHA and EPA, which are crucial to brain and heart health as well as mood stability. Plant sources contain alpha-linolenic acid (ALA), which needs to go through a series of conversions to become DHA and EPA, often inhibited by stress and nutrient deficiencies.

DHA is in high levels in the brain, central nervous system and eyes; EPA supports heart and circulatory functions. Together they have important anti-inflammatory actions in all body cells. Low levels may contribute to weight gain[55] and poor fitness as they help to prevent insulin resistance and degenerative muscle loss, help regulate fats[56] and cholesterol in the liver and bloodstream, help serotonin levels to break craving cycles and help weight loss by improving satiety after meals.[57]

Omega-6 oils are high in the modern diet (from cereals, seed oils and bread) and have been shown to raise levels of endocannabinoids in the brain. Endocannabinoids are substances that repress neurotransmitter release, increasing appetite and dampening memory, mood, pain perception and energy (yep, the same system affected by cannabis and yes, these effects similarly bring on 'the munchies' and are linked to weight gain). Omega-3 oils have shown to reverse these metabolic dysfunctions.[58]

Our hunter-gatherer ancestors probably received 8–12 per cent of their total calories from saturated fat.[59,60] A recent meta-analysis did not support the risk of saturated fats for heart disease, with one study of 53,664 people showing a higher risk of heart attack when saturated fat was replaced by refined carbohydrates.[61] We need a certain amount in our diets to build new cells, to protect organs and for nervous system communication. When levels are low we produce it from carbohydrates, which can lead to sugar cravings. Grass- rather than grain-fed, free-range animals have better fat compositions.

Not all saturated fats behave the same. Plant versions like MCTs (medium-chain triglycerides) in coconuts can't be stored as fat in humans and so act thermogenically, raising fat-burning and metabolism.[62] These are the antibacterial and anti-inflammatory fats like lauric acid and caprylic acid.[63,64,65] also found in human breast milk, pumpkin seeds and butter. Coconut is associated with low obesity and heart disease in cultures that eat it as part of their traditional diet, showing abilities to regulate insulin, prevent metabolic syndrome, reduce heart disease risk factors[66,67] and manage weight.[68]

The replacement of saturated fat with refined vegetable and seed oils has led to an overabundance of omega-6 oils in the modern diet, which is linked to inflammation and heart disease.[69] Removing saturated fat from our diets usually means restricting protein sources and stable fats and replacing them with refined carbohydrates, more polyunsaturated fats (and in refined forms such as trans or hydrogenated fats) and processed foods. Without them we miss a level of appetite satisfaction that can send us towards sugar addiction; vegetarians often crave cheese and chocolate in the winter months, when we need fats for insulation and extra heat production.

Dairy and De-Stress Eating

Dairy is another food that humans have only been eating since we began farming and domesticating animals, but it has become entrenched in our diets through years of recommended intake. We aren't genetically designed to drink milk beyond early infancy, especially not that of another animal. Past the weaning age, most of us naturally lose the ability to digest lactase, the enzyme that breaks down lactose (milk sugar).

It's believed that up to 75 per cent of the world's population is lactose intolerant to some degree,[70] with others probably adapted to produce lactase into adulthood because they are descended from peoples whose earliest ancestors drank milk.[71,72] Lactose has been shown to provoke a high insulin response, and the growth hormones used in mass-farmed dairy products have been implicated in chronic disease, acne and some cancers.[73,74] See more on page 103.

HOW YOU EAT

Without the blood-sugar roller-coaster of a high-sugar diet and stress cravings comes a fantastic feeling of liberation. Becoming more in touch with your energy needs means eating more on some days and less on others at the times that suit your body; like falling into an easy stride.

Mindful eating

Practising mindfulness as you eat will help your digestion and reduce stress-related issues such as bloating – see page 93 for a mindful eating exercise to practise when you need to retune to the quality of your experience. As you eat, ensure you chew every bite slowly – tasting it and savouring it.

Don't skip meals

Although listening to your body's needs is a long-term goal, while making De-Stress changes, not eating can create a blood-sugar dip that kicks the stress response into action and can lead to afternoon and evening binges (especially if it's breakfast you're skipping).[75] Studies have shown that human hunger defaults to three meals a day and that hunger will peak at 7–8 a.m., the most at noon and then 7–8 p.m., even with no knowledge of the time.[76,77] Regular meals help bring other body rhythms into line, which is particularly important for jet-lag recovery, coping with shift work and alleviating Seasonal Affective Disorder.

However, you can vary amounts and times by listening to your body – not cravings – about how much it needs and when. Yes, fasting has health advantages but for the initial six weeks of De-Stress Eating, the priority is to prepare your body so that any periods without food – alongside the usual psycho-social stress of life – can be beneficial and not add to adrenal fatigue. You'll then be able to gauge whether a half- or full-day's fasting feels right and if your blood-sugar levels can cope.

During the initial six weeks of the plan you're encouraged to allow yourself to become hungry *before* you eat. A strong stretch, exercise, craving, lower temperature or hunger pang are good stresses that come with feelings that we often label as 'good' or 'bad'. We have the choice to change our perspective, step away from labelling and feel them just as they are: simply breathe with them, notice they aren't harming us and how they inevitably change and move through. This mindful recalibrating of experience will allow you to connect to your intuition. You'll find answers to the question 'How do I feel?' to guide your changes.

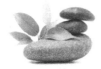

CHAPTER 7

Understanding Cravings

*'If getting upset about something unpleasant is like being
bitten by a snake, grasping for what's pleasant is like
grabbing a snake's tail; sooner or later it will still bite you.'*
AJAHN CHAH

Craving is a sign that we aren't having our needs met. With food, this isn't as simple as nutritional needs, of course: oral gratification can be soothing – just the act of putting things in our mouths can evoke deep body memories of the comforting motion of suckling as a baby.

We're often looking to recreate that rush of the 'love hormone' oxytocin we felt then, and even if we're supplying what most nourishes, satisfies and allows us to best function in the face of stress, there's still stuff we simply 'want' when the going gets tough. All that 'How do I feel?' can quickly translate into 'What will give me a hit?' when we become sad, disappointed, frustrated, angry – all those states that make us want to numb strong and uncomfortable emotions.

The six-week plan in the next chapter will help you enjoy the odd quality treat without resorting to things that just give you a hit and leave you feeling out of control. Recognizing the difference between hunger and craving is a good place to start.

Connect to true hunger

Research from Canada's McMaster University found that 97 per cent of women have felt food cravings as a result of something other than true hunger, and some stress eaters may have lost touch with the feelings of hunger altogether.[1] Real hunger comes on slowly, rarely less than three to five hours after last eating, and is usually accompanied by a hollow feeling in the tummy. It's often satisfied by any palatable food.

Mindless eating is usually done quickly, often as a result of overwhelming feelings, and can manifest as a craving for a specific food. That impulsive 'Ooh, I fancy that' reaction to the sight or smell of tasty food is often false hunger. High levels of sugar and junk fats can desensitize us from natural hunger and food intuition by creating unnatural and addictive body and brain responses.[2]

Anyone who has felt the power of a serious craving for crisps, chocolate or ice cream will know there's something pretty powerful at work. Your brain under stress is in dire need of continual sugar as fuel, and of feel-good chemicals to calm it down, so it seeks out these quick, temporary-fix foods.[3]

In 2006, fascinating research from the University of Michigan in the USA revealed the link between stress and sugar cravings. Researchers presented two groups of rats with sugar pellets and put one group under extreme stress. The stressed-out rats' intensity of bursts of sugar cravings tripled.[4]

Stress is an energy-rich process, demanding an extremely high turnover of the nutrients and fuel we derive from food. But our daily energy production is finite and stress can use up our quota more quickly, as well as nutrients like the B and C vitamins, magnesium and zinc we need for energy and blood-sugar regulation. As stress halts digestion, many of these may be poorly absorbed. Humans particularly crave vitamin C as our main immune protective antioxidant. This means we have a predilection for the sweet taste of ripening fruit, where it's most abundant. As with many things, we've learned to distill out this sweetness and often discard the rest of the fruit, which houses nutrients and fibre that protect us from its harmful effects.

LONG-TERM CHANGE

Liberation from sugar addiction is at the heart of De-Stress Eating, but simply giving up through willpower only to find yourself succumbing to the chocolate mountain at the petrol station isn't a great long-term plan. Understanding the nature of cravings and weaving mindful considerations through our relationships with food can mean that we can stand at that counter and make a conscious decision not to give in – because we know it makes us feel better in the long run.

That doesn't mean we won't have conflict; we simply have too much choice and marketing around us for that to be realistic. But we can develop strategies to notice, breathe and calmly walk away, and not beat ourselves up if that's only *most* of the time!

Emotional attachment to sugar

Our first food, milk, was sweet and then many of us were primed in childhood to see sugar as a source of 'comfort or reward'.[5] When we're stressed we can quickly revert to wanting – and feeling we *deserve* – those comforting or rewarding feelings.[6,7] Changing this perception means accepting that these are only quick-fix solutions that ultimately rob us of sustained energy and a stable mood, while adding to weight gain over the years.

Retraining and liberating

In chapter 9 you can follow the programme to avoid sweet foods for three weeks, so you can desensitize this taste and brain habit. Recent research at Boston University has mapped how the brain can be retrained to enjoy healthy food and decrease sensitivity to the unhealthy, higher-calorie foods when appetite is satisfied by this type of eating.[8]

In the last three weeks of the plan, you can learn to reintroduce select treats to explore how to establish a relationship with sugar that doesn't leave you feeling out of control whenever you get bad news or feel down. That means you can enjoy an ice cream on a summer's day without adding the stress of guilt or fear that it'll spiral you back into old habits.

With De-Stress Eating, we move away from faddy diets in which we label ourselves as 'being good' through willpower, allowing us to connect with a more liberating attitude where healthy is an easy way of life. Using The De-Stress Progress Charts at www.charlottewattshealth.com can help identify craving cycles.

Stress affects hunger and appetite

Studies have demonstrated that high cortisol is associated with increased appetite, and especially cravings for sugar, salt and processed fats, which is why we tend to choose junk or 'comfort' food such as chocolate or crisps when we're under stress.[9] Cortisol influences food consumption by binding to receptors in the brain – specifically the hypothalamus, which governs the HPAA stress response and stimulates appetite for these foods.

Cortisol also indirectly influences appetite by regulating chemicals like CRH (see page 9) and the hormone leptin, which sends a 'stop eating' signal to the brain. High levels of CRH and reduced levels of leptin have been shown to stimulate appetite and a sense of 'need'.[10] Stress can lead us to eat quickly and consume more than we'd like to. The brain's chemical messengers – including 'happy' endorphins and neurotransmitters such as serotonin and dopamine, as well as hormones such as noradrenaline and melatonin – influence how we feel and cope under stress and also help govern what, why, when and how much we eat.

Under chronic stress, their production is dampened, making it hard to tell when you've eaten enough or to attune to body signals. When stress instead of hunger is at the helm of your appetite, you experience blood-sugar imbalances that can turn mindless overeating into a vicious circle.[11,12] Raised cortisol also signals fat to be laid down around the belly, which can add to stress through body image issues.

ADDICTION CYCLES AT WORK

In 2006, scientists used brain-scanning technology to prove that eating junk food is linked to the same emotional reward centres in the brain as those linked to drug addiction.[13,14] When you munch a biscuit, its fats and sugars work on the stressed brain's instinctive need to calm itself down. They signal release of pain-relieving opioids (which sounds like 'opium' for a reason), calming cannabinoids (think cannabis) and serotonin (the body's natural 'happy' chemical) into the brain.

Trouble is, the 'high' never lasts long and is often accompanied by a subsequent mood drop that's worse than when you started out, leaving you hungrier, crankier and craving more of the same. This stress-craving cycle is a type of self-medication, and as with other kinds (cocaine, alcohol and so on), it's habit-forming: the more you do it, the more you want to do it. This habitual stress eating can lead to hard-to-shift weight gain because it becomes your default way of dealing with pressure. And there's *always* pressure.

Sugar is addictive

Sugar addiction fits four of the defined stages of addiction: bingeing, cravings, withdrawal and relapse. Rats given the choice between sugar and cocaine overwhelmingly chose the sugar, even when the cocaine dose offered was raised.

Giving up reliance on sugar as a comfort or reward has many knock-on effects on health. Sugar surges are stimulating in their own right, mimicking the stress response and adding to the agitation and anxiety of 'constant alert'. Excess beyond that which we use as energy is well known to be carcinogenic, inflammatory and ageing.

It's not a matter of willpower

There are two emotional systems at work when we talk about self-control: our impulses and our powers of reflection. Mindful or reflective choices are those made with a sense of creativity, ease and 'take it or leave it'. Impulsive ones are knee-jerk, 'I have to have it now' reactions that are the essence of addictive cycles and self-medication.

If you ever feel in two minds when faced with a tempting something- or someone-or-other, it could be a battle between your impulsive self and your reflective self. These systems compete for control over our reaction or response to some want – be it hunger, lust, rest or whatever. The impulsive self makes fast associations between a choice we face and how it'll make us feel. It scans our environment for quick forms of pleasure and reward. For example, the vending machine equals chocolate equals a sugar hit equals feeling more awake and focused.

Our reflective self, on the other hand, is more concerned with planning, reasoning and long-term goals, such as making a decision to lose weight or get healthy. Studies have found that when we're under stress or have been doing hours of tough mental work, our reflective self is weakened and our impulsive self is more likely to take over, making us less likely to choose what we know will make us feel better long term and more likely to choose the instantly gratifying quick fix.[15] Even if we know full well we might not feel happy about our choice tomorrow, our impulsive self renders us less likely to care in that moment.[16]

When you're stressed and exhausted, your impulsive self seizes the opportunity to take over. Say you've been working long hours for a deadline; once the task is over, the mental strain you've been under makes it less likely you'll be able to resist impulsive, quick gratification like the vending machine, take-away or pub. What strengthens your reflective system is regular, deep rest, relaxation and recovery, *during* stressful times as well as after they have passed.

Evidence shows that regular mindfulness practice strengthens that reflective side throughout all of the food and life choices we make. Over time, prioritizing self-care strengthens your reflective self so it maintains its ability to help you make healthier choices, even under pressure.

MINDFUL EATING

Being fully present while you eat involves sitting and simply eating – being aware of chewing, tasting and savouring every mouthful – not working, walking to the train station, reading, watching TV, surfing the net or walking round the house while talking on the phone. We've become addicted to distraction – the essence of mindlessness – and that's how we end up just ploughing in food we haven't even noticed we've eaten.

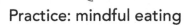

Practice: mindful eating

A mindful eating practice helps us notice how we miss many of the subtleties and richness of a mostly automatic experience. During the following exercise, slow everything right down to truly *feel* your whole body involved in the process:

1. Take a raisin or a nut and place it in the palm of one hand; close your eyes and simply feel its small weight and presence.

2. Look at it from all angles, noticing the colour, shape, texture and size.

3. Feel the weight, texture and any other sensory feedback it gives your sense of touch.

4. Smell it and bring it close to your mouth to introduce it to your body.

5. Put it in your mouth, not chewing yet but just feeling the effects on your tongue and the sensations on the nerves in your mouth. Notice if it's provoking a salivary response.

6. Slowly begin to chew, observing every jaw movement and the effect on the piece of food.

7. Be completely aware of the full spectrum and changing nature of the tastes as the food moves around your mouth and is broken down.

8. Feel your reflex actions carefully, waiting until the optimal time for swallowing, and being aware of the changed taste of the partially digested food.

9. As you swallow, feel the full effects of the food travelling down your throat and the muscular actions that happen automatically.

10. Note how you feel afterwards; the tastes left lingering in your mouth…
are there other sensations?

Mindfulness has been shown to be a useful intervention with eating disorders; in particular, paying attention while eating has a most positive effect on the choice of portion size.[17] So a daily mindfulness meditation practice helps us create a less stressed system to ultimately make better choices, while eating slowly and remaining conscious of the sensory feedback of the tastes and eating process helps us modulate what we eat to what we need.

Disidentification

Mindfulness is becoming accepted as an effective intervention for cravings and addictions of any nature, including smoking, alcohol, drugs and sex.[18] When compared to distracting strategies, the *disidentification* skill that can be practised alongside awareness and acceptance was seen to show success with chocolate cravings.[19]

Disidentification involves seeing the craving as something separate to yourself and viewing it apart to create distance, noticing how you feel away from it. This can also be helpful in noticing the emotional triggers that set off your cravings. Fear is often present and if you disidentify and step aside from it, you can feel that 'awareness of fear is never fearful', as Rick Hanson observes in his book *Buddha's Brain*. If we're not actually running for our lives, chances are we can find a calmer place from which to view our present state.

Mindful preparation for the De-Stress Eating plan

Preparing your landscape to be fully present during this transitional time can make the difference between it feeling like just another fad and laying the foundation for a whole new relationship with your health. Awareness of breath is always the first step – it allows us to find perspective in the calming exhale and a few sighs out can do wonders.

The six-week plan can help you learn an enormous amount about the roots of your habits and craving triggers, but you need to be paying attention to make note of that road map back whenever those periods of stress hit. The times when we wander off and the old habits creep back in… It happens to all of us, but the trick is learning to notice and bring ourselves back without that pesky judgement stealing our energy. Each time it's that much easier – and episodes of turning to the cake or not looking after yourself will become less frequent and severe.

WATCHING NEGATIVE COPING HABITS

When we give up sugar, we may quickly miss the endorphin rush that is the chemical benchmark of addiction. It's easy to transfer this to get a fix from another excessive and consumptive behaviour – shopping, gossiping, excessive exercise, smoking, TV and social networking can all give that buzz, but ultimately they're avoiding the issue of feeling the 'come down'. Building up resources through diet and lifestyle – and embedding healthy endorphin fixes – can free you from this loop. Here's how:

- Be happy and laugh for five minutes, three times a day. Find something or someone that amuses you – a person, a comedy programme on TV or radio – and really let go. This is crucial de-stressing stuff and raises levels of anti-ageing DHEA.

- Spend time nurturing your relationships with others and giving and receiving hugs.

- Exercise – build up to 10 minutes of limbering exercises or stretching, and 45 to 50 minutes of brisk walking.

- Enjoy sex – even fun sexual fantasies raise endorphins.

- Sing and dance – there's an exhilarating reason why choirs and Zumba have become so popular recently. Dance around your home!

- Be outside for one hour per day, especially if you work indoors and/or are exposed to a lot of electronic equipment – computers, printers, cars, planes, etc.

- Be aware of all the ways that you consume: not just food, but also stuff you buy, information you take in and stimuli you've become used to. Only buying what you need (not want), being mindful of information that causes you distress and watching when you turn to

TV, internet shopping or Twitter as a distraction can help to diminish time spent supplying the stimulation that triggers food cravings.

- Practise compassion and do the Metta Bhavana meditation on page 189 to raise dopamine levels and reduce the need to spike them with quick fixes.

Intercepting cravings on the go

Having simple tools to draw you back to a place of calm and presence can be the difference between running to the cake shop and retaining some sense of control:

- Make a fist to represent feeling stressed or craving. Release a finger to say the following affirmations to draw you back to a reflective state. Thumb: 'I notice how I feel'; index finger: 'I accept myself'; third finger: 'I calm myself'; ring finger: 'I notice how I feel now'; little finger: 'I'm healthy and happy.' Then open your hand to say, 'My open hand represents calm and relaxation.' You can change these to any positive phrases in the present tense that work for you.

- Place coloured dot stickers (or any shape that works for you) around the house, for example, behind the kettle or on the fridge door, to remind yourself to pause and be in the present for a few breaths. This can programme in the priority to slow down, to feel and move away from the tendencies to rush through life that send signals to fuel up that express as cravings. You can then add these reminders wherever helps – your desk, purse, diary – anywhere you look often and can access as you need to.

Supplementing De-Stress Eating

We live in a world where the nutrients we need aren't available in food because of poor soil and large-scale farming practices, and we quickly use up those we do absorb in response to stress, pollution and medications. Visit www.charlottewattshealth.com for the free De-Stress Supplement Guide for sources of nutrients commonly deficient in those with cravings and addictive cycles.

CHAPTER 8

De-Stress Eating Basics

'If you don't look after your body, where are you going to live?'
UNKNOWN

Connecting with the what, how and when you eat is the basis of De-Stress Eating. The six-week plan is designed to help you explore and ask 'How do I feel?' at every point – to understand what best feeds your optimal capacity to feel calm, supported and free from stress caused by food itself. This will help if you've been feeling:

- Unsure of how best to support energy and protect your body from the effects of stress
- Controlled by cravings, urges and appetite
- That you don't understand what suits you and feel confusion around food and your body responses
- That your relationship with food is disordered and problematic

Advice to eat 'little and often' or snacking habits can have us automatically putting something in our mouths at the slightest itch of hunger. Hunger pangs are just like any other good stress: challenges (like a strong stretch, exercise, a craving or lowered temperature) that come with feelings that we often label 'good' or 'bad'.

The odd night out or an irresistible tiramisu don't matter in the scheme of things when you default to a lifestyle that supports your body systems towards minimizing stress responses and balancing blood sugar. De-Stress Eating isn't confined to what you put in your mouth at a meal, but is viewed within the larger context of your daily life.

If you're regularly incorporating mindfulness and mindful movement into your everyday routine, and avoiding sugar and refined carbohydrates *most of the time*, you have the freedom to enjoy the odd deviation without guilt, knowing that your body will handle it much better than it would if you were in a more stressed state.

THE SIX-WEEK PLAN

To help you get back in touch with your natural hunger, relationship and rhythm with food, the De-Stress Eating six-week plan is divided into two phases:

Weeks 1–3: Retraining taste. As you move away from the habits that keep you in addictive and fat-storing cycles you'll reconnect to natural hunger signals. You'll develop changing tastes and move away from craving sugar, salt and junk fats towards a calmer, healthier relationship with food.

Weeks 4–6: Food liberation. As you feel more connected and trusting of your instincts, you'll probably notice your appetite and sense of hunger are guided by your energy levels instead of your stress. Increased sensitivity to how certain foods and drinks make you feel will help you explore what suits *you*.

Below are the basic guidelines for what to eat on the De-Stress Eating six-week plan. You can also use the De-Stress Progress Charts at www. charlottewattshealth.com as motivational tools.

Protein

This should make up a quarter or a third of each meal.

- Animal protein in the form of eggs, meat, fish and shellfish make the foundation of the kind of meal our ancestors would have eaten, to which you can add twice as many vegetables, both as salads and cooked.

- The starchy carbohydrate or grain part can be avoided, or varied to suit individual needs, with a daily portion of well-cooked beans the best choice.

- For vegetarians, protein in the form of nuts, seeds, live full-fat yoghurt and goat's cheese can be added to salads and to stir-fries or roast vegetables for quick meals.

- Vegans, see page 129 for how to prepare grains and beans safely for higher intake.

Plenty of vegetables

Aim for six to eight palm-sized portions each day.

- Raw salad vegetables provide fibre and key nutrients. Have them with a tablespoon or two of cold-pressed extra virgin olive oil to absorb fat-soluble nutrients like vitamins A, E and beta carotene.[1]

- Have as many cooked vegetables as raw; these are easier to digest.

- Dark green leafy vegetables and bitter salad leaves like spinach, watercress and radicchio should be eaten liberally.

- Have cruciferous vegetables at least four times a week, daily when possible. These include broccoli, cabbage, kale, pak choi, mustard leaves and Brussels sprouts. Avoid eating these raw, though, as they interfere with thyroid function.

- Roots that can be eaten raw for some starch energy include carrots, radishes and grated beetroot.

- Garlic and onions can be eaten in abundance.

- Eat seaweeds for iodine and other minerals (see page 59).

- Eat as many brightly coloured veg as possible, for antioxidant variety.

- Don't rely on the nightshade family of vegetables, as these are high in inflammatory lectins (see page 62). Eat tomatoes, peppers, potatoes and aubergines sparingly, cooking them to reduce their lectin content.

Healthy fats

- Omega oils or polyunsaturated fats should make up the main part of your fat intake, especially omega-3 oils from oily fish such as sardines, mackerel, wild salmon and trout as well as eggs and meat from grass- (not grain-) fed free-range animals.

- Monounsaturated Fatty Acids or MUFAs from avocados, almonds, olives and olive oil, nuts and seeds should be included wherever possible.

- Vegans should include coconut, peanuts, Brazil nuts, cashews, pumpkin seeds and pine nuts for vital saturated fats.

- Use unrefined, cold-pressed oils such as olive, flax and sesame oil for dressings.

- Use coconut oil, olive oil or butter to cook with.

Alkalizing foods

- Vegetables, fruit, seeds, herbs and spices help keep us in the slightly alkaline blood pH levels at which the body works best. This helps balance acidity from stress, grains, beans and animal produce.

- Almonds, coconut, sesame seeds, chestnuts and pine nuts are alkaline (other nuts are acidic so balance out with veg).

- Add lemon juice to water and dressings.

Liver-supporting foods

- Eat sulphur-rich foods such as watercress, garlic, onions, leeks and fennel for liver detoxification.

- Cruciferous vegetables (above) contain sulforaphane chemicals that enable you to produce antioxidant enzymes in the liver that work over and over again long after eating and are anti-inflammatory.[2,3]

- Turmeric, green tea, avocados, raspberries and oily fish all help liver function.

Bitter foods

- Use endive, radicchio, chicory, romaine or cos lettuce and watercress in salads. Their bitter taste stimulates digestive juices.

- Have bitter foods such as olives, grapefruit or bitter leaves before your main meal – these are classic starter ingredients and help us get the best nutrition from our food, resulting in fewer cravings to make up deficits.

- Lemon juice in hot water first thing in the morning wakes up digestion and appetite, and between meals it keeps us alkalized.

Fresh fruit

- Eat whole: two to three pieces a day maximum.

- Drink less fruit juice (or avoid it) and eat fruit raw and whole wherever you can. Although it's rich in nutrients and great eaten in moderation, fruit is also high in sugars (especially modern varieties) and can keep a sweet tooth alive (see best sweet alternatives on pages 167–68).

Drink adequate fluids

Have non-sugary, non-caffeinated drinks in between meals, as thirst dictates; choices include fresh, pure water, herbal or green tea and plenty of vegetables and fruit.

Wean yourself off sugar and processed foods

The more you look after what you do put into your body – and prioritize De-Stress lifestyle advice – the more you'll be able easily and successfully to handle tapering off sugars, stimulants and the sugar/fat combinations that your brain may have become used to receiving during stressful periods. See chapter 7 (Understanding Cravings) and modify the following foods to help regulate insulin production.

What to avoid

- Processed fats low in omega-3 oils – vegetable and seed oils (especially for cooking), poor-quality spreads (use butter or olive oil instead), cheap meat and eggs, commercial mayonnaises and dressings.

- Poor-quality meat, eggs and fish – unhealthy fats from sedentary, poorly fed animals that pass their bad luck on to you; processed meats like salami or those cured with nitrates. Pay more money and cut back on convenience or junk foods and things you don't need – with less stress you'll find that comfort buying lessens and you can redirect money to nourish yourself more. You'll also be supporting ethical animal farming, a compassionate approach (see www.ciwf.org.uk).

- Sugar and processed junk – sugar in all its forms, sweeteners, damaged fats, ready meals, take-away food; ingredients that sound more like chemicals than food are just that.

What to limit or avoid

- Grains/cereals – wheat, rye, oats, barley flour, bran, quinoa, rice, corn, maize, all flours and 'milks' from these.

- Beans/legumes and pulses – beans (soy, pinto, chickpea, mung, aduki, black, cannellini, etc.), peas, green beans, French beans, peanuts, ground nuts, pine nuts, flours like soy flour, gram flour, lentil flour in poppadoms, all flours and 'milks' from these.

- Roots that need cooking – potatoes, sweet potatoes, parsnips, yams, cassava, tapioca.

- Dairy – whole and skimmed milk, cheap cheese, fruit yoghurts and processed powdered milk forms.

Starchy carbohydrates

During the first phase of the De-Stress Eating plan, finding the right balance of grains, beans, starchy roots (such as potatoes and yams) and dairy can help insulin levels and appetite satisfaction. For some people these foods can cause bloating, tiredness and indigestion as well as weight gain. If that's you, cutting these foods could lead to effortless weight loss where needed, more energy and relief from post-lunch bloating.

For others, avoiding these starches leaves them feeling listless, as though something is missing from their diets. During the first three weeks of this plan you'll be able to decide if your individual chemistry responds best to a diet that includes small amounts of grains and beans cooked in the best way.

So, unless you're a vegetarian (and may need the protein from beans), during the first three weeks of the plan avoid grains and beans and take note of your energy levels. If you feel great and your stress symptoms, energy and weight improve, you may not handle them well. If you find your energy levels lower, introduce one serving a day of beans at breakfast or lunch in the fourth week. In chapter 10 you'll find instructions for cooking your grains in safe and healthy ways.

DAIRY AND THE FLEXI-PALEO DIET

Our ancestors didn't eat dairy but got their calcium (with magnesium) from green leaves, nuts and fish; with plenty of weight-bearing exercise and sunlight, this kept their bones strong. During the plan, avoid dairy or reduce your intake to an organic serving or two every two to four days.[4] If you're a vegetarian you may need to include a little more well-chosen dairy in your diet, ensuring probiotic levels are good to help you digest it.[5]

- Greek feta cheese from grass-fed goat's milk has a better fat profile than an average commercial cheddar or Swiss cheese. Feta has much lower saturated fat and contains omega-3 oils not found in cow's milk cheeses, making it healthier than a low-fat cheddar.

- Goat's and sheep's milk products contain smaller lactose (milk sugar) molecules than cow's, so are easier to digest.

- Greek yoghurt contains less sugar and more protein than regular yoghurt, as it's sieved to remove the carbohydrate-rich whey. Its thickness leaves you fuller for longer (you may need less) than more watery versions and the lower lactose – milk sugar – makes it easier to digest. It is also more delicious!

- Hard cheese and butter have lower lactose levels, so a lower insulin response than milk and cream. So, a slither or two of hard cheese every few days and a pat of organic butter on your vegetables are good choices, but remember, these are high in saturated fat so balance with other fats in oily fish, olives, olive oil, nuts and seeds.

- Full-fat dairy is preferable to skimmed or low-fat, which is processed, less satisfying and lacks fat-soluble nutrients (important for lactose-tolerant vegetarians); full-fat has also been shown to be better for weight loss. Without fat the liver struggles to handle the protein from milk.

A2 milk proteins are best

These are the genetic form of the beta casein milk protein molecule best tolerated by humans and were present in all dairy herds until a natural mutation in European herds thousands of years ago. The more modern A1 protein is believed to be linked to intolerance and conditions such as asthma, eczema, hayfever and IBS.[6,7]

Today, cow's milk mostly has a mixture of the two, with only certified Jersey and Guernsey cows producing A2 milk, which is stated on labels. Milk from goats, sheep, camels, buffalo, yaks and donkeys is mostly or completely A2.

CHAPTER 9

Six Weeks to De-Stress Eating

'Today you are You, that is truer than true.
There is no one alive who is Youer than You.'
DR SEUSS

WEEKS 1–3: RETRAINING TASTE

The best time to start this first phase of the plan is when you can have enough space to look after yourself – perhaps a weekend when no one is coming to stay and you've no other commitments. Remember, you're looking to explore what works for you, for life, not to avoid things through gritted teeth for a short period of time.

We all have blips in life, so if you don't live up to your ideal all the time, be kind to yourself and simply start again the next day. As positive factors increase, the pull of the negatives will decrease and more balanced biochemistry will take the place of willpower.

Regulating blood-sugar balance can take time after years of irregularities, and you may initially have a period of adjustment where you crave sugar and refined foods more as your brain chemistry readjusts.[1] Practise mindfulness regularly to sit with any discomfort that cravings produce – simply feeling them expansively to get out of the grip of needing to react.

Let me know the day you're starting your De-Stress Eating at www.charlottewattshealth.com and you'll be sent supporting emails to provide extra motivation and well-timed tips along your journey.

Moving away from stress-inducing foods

In these first three weeks, focus on avoiding the following foods:

- High-sugar/high-GI foods – processed cereals, refined 'white' grains, soft drinks, fruit juices, added sugars, confectionery, sweets, chocolate, fruit-flavoured products, low-fat desserts including frozen yoghurt, alcohol

- High-sugar/high-'bad' fat combination foods – ice cream, cakes, biscuits, pastries, cheap bread, pasties, sausage rolls, desserts with dairy and sugar, custard, cheap dark chocolate, any milk chocolate, commercial sandwiches

- Gluten and dairy – those with digestive and immune responses to gluten in wheat, rye and barley (also oats if processed in the same factory as gluten-containing foods) and dairy may find that the chemical rush these might bring can set off sugar cravings, so it's worth avoiding them fully for these three weeks. If you're a vegetarian, see the dairy guidelines on page 103.

- Stimulants – alcohol, caffeine, nicotine, recreational drugs. If you have addictions to any of these, address sugar and stress issues in preparation for giving them up, but you do need to be ready, so plan into weeks 4–6, or give yourself a realistic goal for a later date.

How sugar hides in food labels

Sugar is sugar, and saying it's 'natural' or organic does not change its effects in the body – if it tastes sweet, it is. Increasing exercise is no reason to increase sugar intake; higher activity means a higher need for protective antioxidants – and excess sugar impedes muscle performance and strength.

Sports nutrition products can be high in sugars, while natural fruit, nuts and coconut water provide more supportive fuel. Manufacturers use many ways to hide the sugar content of foods – see the list of sugars below, which are often seen in 'fruit-flavoured' products, even 'natural', organic ones:

- agave syrup
- barley malt
- beet sugar
- brown rice syrup
- brown sugar
- cane juice
- corn sweetener
- corn syrup
- date sugar
- demerara sugar
- dextrin
- maltose
- mannitol, sorbitol, xylitol
- maple syrup
- microcrystalline cellulose
- molasses
- maltodextrin

- unrefined sugar
- white sugar
- polydextrose
- raisin juice
- raw sugar
- sucrose
- dextrose
- fructose (from fruit and grains)
- fruit juice concentrate
- galactose (from milk)
- glucose
- granulated sugar
- high-fructose corn syrup
- honey
- invert sugar
- lactose (from milk)
- malted barley

Natural sugars

Natural fruit sugars like fructose (e.g. in agave syrup) and date sugar aren't better because they appear to come from plants (all sugars do, except lactose in milk). Fructose is more difficult than sucrose (table sugar) for our bodies to process. Although causing less of a rise in blood sugar, fructose can raise blood triglycerides (fats), contribute to weight gain, affect mood and rob the liver of energy when it's eaten outside the safer package of a whole fruit.[2,3]

Honey is the only sugar source our ancestors would have eaten, but only occasionally. It has a lower Glycaemic Index (GI) than refined sugar, but it's still high in fructose, so use it sparingly and pay more for antibacterial Manuka honey.

Artificial sweeteners and sweet-taste withdrawal

Sweeteners are often added to products to enable them to be labelled as 'diet' or 'low sugar', but this isn't a healthier option. The science and evidence remains unclear about sweeteners, but remember they are big business and are designed to cause a response in the brain. Aspartame, for instance, a common sweetener in 'diet' products, sweets and soft drinks (as brands Nutrasweet and Equal), has recently been shown to raise glucose levels in people with diabetes.[4]

Sweeteners aren't 'free calories', they come with a price – keeping a sweet tooth and cravings alive. They are often found in highly processed foods that upset our biochemistry – it's much better to save a sweet taste and occasionally go for a better-quality chocolate or pudding as a treat.

When our brains are told we've eaten something sweet but then don't receive the calories, this can confuse appetite regulation and actually raise it.[5] If you use sugar or sweeteners in tea or coffee, don't find substitutes, instead wean yourself off – a sweet tooth is quickly changed.

Be prepared for sugar withdrawal effects such as headaches, irritability, anger, energy slumps, depression and fatigue within this first phase of the plan.[6] In some people these can last for weeks, but many others report feeling great pretty quickly, once these initial symptoms have subsided.

Get sugar savvy

Anything over 10g (½oz) of sugar per 100g (3½oz) on a label is too much, and with a processed food that can equate to sugars that raise blood sugar and turn to fat. A can of sweet fizzy drink contains around four teaspoons of sugar.[7]

Sugar-craving solutions

Giving up sugar 'cold turkey' can initially lead to poor glucose supply to the brain, which causes poor serotonin regulation and a subsequent drop in mood. This can happen around three or four days after giving up sugar and can lead to binges and cravings. This is temporary and will pass as your system gets used to slower-release forms of fuel to the body and brain, but you may want to time this for over a weekend if you know you have an ingrained sugar habit.

Use the sugar-weaning tips on page 95, along with the following suggestions for lasting change:

- We typically have a blood sugar low at 4 p.m. when traditionally the tea and cakes were wheeled out. If this is your point of least resistance, eat a healthy snack at this time or just before. Although less snacking overall is the ideal scenario, it's preferable to choose a better snack at the right time than mainline the sugar later. See chapter 12 for more on De-Stress drinks and snacks.

- Constant cravings for sugar can indicate that there aren't enough healthy, good-quality proteins and fats in your diet, as these register satisfaction in the brain, whereas carbohydrates do not. Be particularly aware of this if you're a vegetarian or (especially) a vegan.

- Xylitol is the best sugar substitute choice, with some positive effects seen on weight loss, but it can still keep a sweet tooth alive.[8] Substitute it for sugar in tea or coffee, then wean yourself off it bit by bit over a few weeks.

- Use natural, slow-release sugars that provide a sweet taste, like unsweetened coconut, ground almond, natural vanilla essence and unsweetened apple puree. Coconut contains plant-saturated fats called medium-chain triglycerides (MCTs) that help satisfy any need for sugar as they provide a dense energy source (see page 84). Use as unsweetened desiccated coconut or flakes.

- Use cinnamon as much as possible: it contains a bioflavonoid called MHCP (methylhydroxychalcone polymer) that mimics insulin, actively moving sugar into cells for energy and sensitizing insulin receptors.[9]

A teaspoon a day helps balance blood-sugar levels in people with diabetes. It's highly effective at telling the brain that you've eaten something sweet, with positive rather than negative consequences. Add it to coffee, tea, yoghurt, berries, curries, and see spice teas on page 172.

- A small portion of starchy carbs, such as new potatoes or sweet potatoes, can be included at dinner if you're suffering late-night binges. You can then wean yourself off this as you regulate energy and cravings while giving up refined sugars.[10]

- If you really need a sweet hit, choose a banana – they calm by helping levels of the anti-anxiety neurotransmitter gamma-aminobutyric acid (GABA) and serotonin. Full-fat plain yoghurt with banana, cinnamon and coconut can satisfy extreme cravings if you're weaning yourself off desserts.

Natural detoxification

'Detox' doesn't refer only to a specialized cleansing ritual – it's a natural process that occurs in every one of your cells, tissues and organs continually. It's like breathing: as long as you're taking in air, water, food and substances from the environment, you'll need to clear out by-products. Getting wastes out of cells allows nutrients in and relies on the right foods, less stress, circulation through movement, better breathing and fresh air.

You're likely to feel the effects of detoxification within these first few days to weeks of the plan. This will depend on your liver capacity and previous habits. Side effects are signs that you're making a positive difference and that there may be backed-up toxins circulating in your bloodstream.

Every aspect of The De-Stress Effect helps improve detoxification. This may be seen as skin eruptions, fatigue and headaches, but also revisiting of any symptoms you tend to experience. Women may have one difficult menstrual cycle before monthly cycles and PMS improve. Many people go through a period where this release can lead to revisiting past emotions, which they may feel they need to address and hold with kind attention.

Stress reduces the liver's ability to break down toxins and balance hormones, so lifestyle measures are crucial to managing these cycles on many levels. Liver function is at the heart of balancing blood sugar and reducing cravings. You can provide extra help with the following:

- Hydration (see page 170).
- Liver-supporting foods (see page 100).
- Circulation: outdoor walks, yoga and breathing exercises keep blood flow and lymphatic movement fluid.
- Massage, saunas and steams: these help calm nerves, lower stress hormones and release toxins in muscles and through skin.
- Dry skin-brushing: the friction from dry brush bristles increases circulation and draws toxins out towards the skin, as well as creating a 'good stress' that wakes up immunity to the outside of the body. Buy a not-too-soft body brush with all natural bristles and before a bath or shower, brush your whole body in long strokes towards the heart.
- Epsom salts or Dead Sea salts baths: use a cupful to help release tight muscles (including the bowel) and to detoxify. Stay in the bath for 20 minutes but don't have the water too hot (the brave can have a cold shower afterwards for a 'good stress' sauna/spritz effect).
- Ayurvedic oils: use after a bath or shower. Before drying, quickly rub unrefined organic sesame or linseed oil straight onto skin. This is an ancient Ayurvedic practice that works wonders for circulation.

Weight loss

The plan will support weight loss if it's needed. You may lose more weight in the first week than in any other, as you shed fluid through the first stage of detoxification. If you must weigh yourself, do it only once a week, with 0.5–1kg (1–2lb) a week the healthiest speed for dropping any excess and keeping it off. Bodies naturally plateau, as they easily adapt to any new situation, so stick with it when weight loss seems to come to a halt: it will pick up again if you continue with dietary changes and exercise.

Keep on moving

At least one daily bowel movement is crucial for eliminating the day's toxins and metabolic wastes, but also for regulating hormones, cholesterol and immunity. If you experience constipation, follow the liver support advice above, increasing soluble fibre through vegetables, nuts and fruit, and ensuring good bowel hydration with the measures on page 171. You can also try the following:

- Exercise: squatting motions and abdominal exercises stimulate peristalsis, the movement of muscles in the gut; these muscles need daily toning as much as any other.

- Yoga breathing and postures help the gut move and relax, especially twists, which massage the intestines.

- Bircher muesli (see page 136) with extra prunes and/or unsulphured dried apricots added and soaked in, or with added stewed plums, apples and soaked linseeds, will have a natural laxative effect.

- Extra help at www.charlottewattshealth.com in the De-Stress Supplement Guide

Realistic, steady, lifelong change

From sugary snacks to pizza, the fewer of your 'habit foods' you have, the easier it gets and you'll soon see your tastes change. It can take just days for a sweet tooth to decrease and for sugary foods to start to taste overly sweet. So stick with it and the foods you may think you can't live without may suddenly seem less appealing.

Three meals a day and no snacks are the De-Stress recommendation – the right meal at the right time should be able to sustain blood sugar for the four to five hours until the next meal and allow for full digestion and natural signs of hunger in between. If needed, a well-timed snack can help curb cravings for sugar at other times; see chapter 14 for suggestions.

Sugar, salt and chemical flavourings can numb taste buds so that subtle tastes such as those of herbs and vegetables seem bland. These substances also alter brain chemistry and the way we respond to foodstuffs. During this first phase of the plan you'll be changing your palate and tasting more subtle and sophisticated flavours so you can enjoy healthier foods.

Troubleshooting

Problem: You suffer from sugar cravings.

Solution: Too few fats or protein in your diet could be the cause, so ensure you're eating enough of these to satisfy your appetite. Note any differences in sugar cravings without the presence of starches in your diet. Some may find they disappear altogether, others may find they crave sugar for energy.

If you're in the latter group, try a daily portion of either sourdough rye bread or soaked oats in the Bircher muesli at breakfast (see page 136) or beans, new potatoes or a sweet potato at lunch for a few days. Experiment with these choices and if you still need help satisfying cravings as you move away from sugar, you may need a portion at both meals.

Problem: You have the urge to binge.

Solution: Those who tend towards overeating or binge eating can be set off by the insulin surge from grains, beans, potatoes, sweet potatoes – and of course refined sugars, stimulants and stress hormones. If you're in this camp, cutting these out entirely may help reinstate the satiety hunger 'off switch'.

Problem: You don't feel satisfied without something sweet after lunch.

Solution: Be assured that this tendency is a mind and body conditioning that can change. Reduce sugars elsewhere in your diet and follow the recommendations on page 109 to move away from sugar. Have a herbal tea with liquorice and/or cinnamon to help regulate insulin and tell your brain you've received something sweet. A portion of berries is the best sweet choice as a dessert.

Problem: You crave comfort carbs such as sweet foods and salty snacks at night.

Solution: Before you comfort eat, ask yourself, 'What's this about?' Do you feel angry, tired or wired? Is there something – other than what you're about to eat – that might help more? If your comfort is sitting in front of the television and eating something numbing, find other ways to soothe yourself. If you fancy food comfort in the form of creamy pasta or crisps, your body might simply be craving calming fats. Good fats such as avocado, a knob of butter, chopped nuts or pine nuts added to vegetables can help satisfy that urge and provide a feeling of calm without the excess salt, junk fats and blood-sugar spikes.

If you feel wired and manic, your body may be craving comfort food simply to calm down. Try a salt bath before bed for immediate calm to your muscles and mind, but let yourself cool down before sleep or the temperature change can cause waking. Replace crisps with pumpkin or sunflower seeds, which are rich in the amino acid tryptophan, from which your body makes mood-enhancing serotonin. If you're craving salt, this may be due to flagging adrenal glands, so try adding good-quality rock salt to your dinner.

WEEKS 4–6: FOOD LIBERATION

By now you'll have an understanding, through personal experience, of how the food you choose and the lifestyle choices you make affect the way you feel and look. This 'sense memory' and intuition are more powerful than anything you could read.[11] It's likely you'll also be moving your life to a more balanced place as the nutrition, relaxation and lifestyle practices outlined here and in previous chapters have an impact on your stress levels and mood.

For some people this can take longer as they settle into new ways of shopping and understanding healthy food choices and cooking, but it all helps you understand and trust what suits you.

In this second phase of the De-Stress Eating plan, the main change is the option to introduce occasional treats like alcohol or chocolate to your diet. Unrealistic and over-regimented diets don't work in the long term, so these three weeks are about setting the scene for true change and deciding what will work for you on a daily basis.

Stay flexible to avoid stress being created if it all goes awry – you can always pull back to abstinence to clear the decks whenever you need to. The most important part of the plan is allowing change to settle and take effect. Weeks 4–6 are about observing how the changes make you feel, learning what works for you (and what doesn't!) and what you'll take with you into the rest of your life.

Treats and habits – learning the difference

If blood-sugar balance is regulated our bodies can handle the odd spike. To achieve this you need to be clear about the difference between a treat and a habit:

- A treat is something that you enjoy occasionally – it gives you pleasure, but you don't feel controlled by it; yes, you deserve it now and then, but you're aware that, ultimately, it works against your health goals.

- A habit is something you eat or drink regularly – every day or few days – even feeling it 'normalizes' you.

- If eating a food you consider a treat makes you feel guilty, or as if you're failing, ask yourself whether it's creeping in as a habit or if you're being too hard on yourself.

It can be easier when you have a strict no-go policy on the so-called 'baddies', but this can become another source of psycho-social stress for those who don't like rules or authority. If complete avoidance of the odd treat works for you, identify and accept that. If you need to know you can have that indulgence two or three times a week or you'll rebel and eat the whole cake shop, know that too and plan the best way to do it.

Quality not quantity

Pick your treats based on quality, not quantity. For example, a few quality chocolate Brazil nuts rather than a bar of dodgy milk chocolate. High-quality foods are often more satisfying; what's the point of a treat that you don't fully enjoy? Or if wine is your thing, better quality and half as much can help you savour it.

Stop before you hit the point where you feel 'dirty', and find the stage where you can control cravings but not deny yourself, so you don't feel the need to rebel but are moving away from feeling confused or neurotic around food. Other examples of quality treats include a small cup of gourmet ice cream or a small serving of homemade pudding. You get the idea.

A bean/grain plan

By now you'll have worked out whether cutting out grains and beans entirely works for you or whether one or two servings a day suits you better. If you choose to include whole grains and beans, avoid them at dinner, when your body doesn't need them to fuel activity. If you're a vegetarian, stick to one serving of grains and one of beans, but not at the same meal. For most non-vegetarians, one portion of grains and/or beans maximum daily is ample, especially if outweighed by vegetables, good protein and healthy fats.

During weeks 4–6, revisit the troubleshooting suggestions on page 113 when needed and consider:

- If you want to lose weight – replace grains, beans and potatoes with vegetables, nuts and seeds. Remember that these are still carbohydrate plant foods, but have more soluble than insoluble fibre for greater appetite control. A recent study showed that by increasing soluble fibre by just 10g (0.4oz) a day, 3.7 per cent of dangerous deep belly fat was reduced over a five-year period.[12]

- If you've been eating some grains, beans or potatoes to help with sugar withdrawal – you may now be able to explore removing them to monitor craving or binge cycles.

- If you want to include beans/grains and are vegetarian or vegan – your best choice is a slice of sourdough rye bread or soaked oats in the Bircher muesli (see page 136) at breakfast or a small portion of well-cooked beans, new potatoes or sweet potato at lunch. Always eat with vegetables (or fruit if Bircher muesli) for vitamin C to help reduce anti-nutrients and absorb iron.

- If you experience constipation – this might result from reducing the amount of insoluble fibre you'd normally get from grains and beans, even while increasing soluble fibre levels in vegetables, fruit and nuts. See the 'Keep on moving' section of this chapter. If this doesn't improve things in a fortnight, add one to two portions of whole grains and beans.

Healthy grain guidelines

If you decide to include grains in your diet, avoid cheap, commercial breads and choose instead small bakery and sourdough loaves. Also avoid raw grains in muesli and unfermented soy in soy milk and flour. Switch to rye where possible, as it contains less gluten than wheat and helps iron and zinc absorption. Sourdough rye bread is the best choice, as the fermentation with the lactic acid rye naturally contains breaks down gluten more.[13,14] Similarly, soaking oats in lactic-acid-containing yoghurt for Bircher muesli makes them more digestible.

Avoid wheat, to give your digestion and immune system a break from gluten. Even if you're not intolerant it will help your beneficial gut bacteria and this may positively impact your serotonin levels and mood.

Find your personal grain tolerance levels by avoiding foods you react to (with spots round the mouth, bloating, wind or tiredness) or keeping your intake occasional. You may see that you can handle fewer grains and beans when you're stressed – often, ironically, the times when you're not able to make the best choices (for example, that dodgy sandwich at the airport after a long-haul flight). The more you can help yourself with better choices when they're available, the less you'll react to the exceptions.

Addictions

If you have addictive patterns to other substances, such as caffeine beyond a couple of cups a day, alcohol, cigarettes or recreational drugs, consider at what stage you now see yourself with lowered influence of chronic stress, sugar, refined carbohydrates and excess junk fats.

Be careful not to increase your intake of other addictive substances to replace sugar, so that from there you can plan when you might feel is the right time to give up. Continuing with the De-Stress Eating and lifestyle tools will help you create the energy and brain chemicals that will make giving up these other things far easier.[15,16]

Reviewing your progress

You might want to revisit any of the following to give yourself some perspective on where you are and where you're heading. After all, you're unravelling years of stressful living and are just at the beginning:

The Stress Gauge (see pages 4–7)
The Stress Suits (see chapter 5)
De-Stress Eating Principles (see chapter 6)
De-Stress Reflection Journal (see pages 251–52)

See www.charlottewattshealth.com to download these, the De-Stress Progress Charts and others for repeated use.

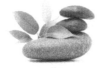

CHAPTER 10

The Building Blocks of Healthy Eating

*'One cannot think well, love well, sleep
well, if one has not dined well.'*
VIRGINIA WOOLF

There's no hidden secret to healthy cooking. Once you know a few simple principles it can be less complicated than 'unhealthy' cooking, and dishes can often be thrown together in almost the same time it takes to peel the plastic off a ready meal to heat it up.

This chapter is designed to give you the simple strategies you need to make the healthy cooking basics – stews, salads and stir-fries – more effortless. There are no defined weights or calories included and counting or measuring food beyond rough volumes is avoided. This might make serial dieters feel uncertain at first, but it is a good way to foster a healthy sense of liberation around food.

Allowing yourself to connect with natural appetite, hunger and fullness signals is a crucial part of the De-Stress process. Don't worry about getting 'out of control' around the food. As you're avoiding trigger foods such as sugars, junk fats and refined carbohydrates, as well as identifying your stress cravings and false hunger, your body will begin to connect with the amounts it needs on different days.

If you're used to having lots of salt or sugary foods, it might take some time for your taste buds to acclimatize to new tastes, but after a few weeks you'll be appreciating more subtle and sophisticated flavourings.

Start experimenting and using cooking as one of your meditative activities, staying present and perhaps listening to relaxing music as you chop and prepare. You might have the odd slightly strange outcome, but that's the worst that can happen. If you're already a whizz in the kitchen, there's plenty to explore in the suggestions below to find the healthiest foods that suit your palate. Add your own twists and note favourite combinations to build a repertoire that encourages variety.

The following chart gives information on the sources and quantities of the best foods to buy and use as the basis of your meals. You can make a shopping list of these, according to your taste preferences and what you are using for the cooking suggestions in this chapter. Quantities shown are per person, per meal. See pages 98–101 for details of how to include them in your daily diet.

Sources and quantities		
Ingredient	Amount per person	Healthy option
Vegetables	At least one handful of three or more kinds per day.	Organic where possible, see www.ewg. org/foodnews/list/ for foods to prioritize to lower your pesticide load.
Meat	One palm-sized piece; prioritize quality over quantity and you may find you're satisfied with less.	Free-range, organic, grass-fed meat including game, liver and other organ meats where possible.[1] If wild or pasture-raised animal products are hard to obtain, beef and lamb are the best domesticated choices; cured meats (bacon, ham) no more than once or twice a week.[2]
Fish – oily	A palm-sized piece, two to three times a week maximum, to avoid toxic build-up	Sustainable, mercury-free wild fish: Alaskan salmon, mackerel, sardines, herring, anchovies, trout; avoid mercury-high tuna, swordfish and marlin.[3,4]
Fish – white and seafood	A palm-sized piece; this is a good substitute for red meat	Sustainable and mercury-free sources: line-caught pollock, halibut, haddock; farmed clams, scallops, squid, prawns, shrimp.

(continued)

Sources and quantities		
Ingredient	Amount per person	Healthy option
Eggs	One to two per day	From free-range, organic, grass-fed chickens where possible; free-range at the very least.
Dairy	Occasional small block of feta or other cheese, if tolerant. One tablespoon Greek live or full-fat live or 'bio' yoghurt, if tolerant (see dairy info on page 103)	Prioritize organic where possible to avoid high levels of hormones and antibiotics[5] and for healthier fat profile.[6]
Beans/ legumes/ pulses	Half a mug cooked volume – according to tolerance (see page 102)	Organic, darker coloured varieties, such as black beans, are higher in antioxidants.
Nuts	One palmful maximum daily, in meals or as a snack	Organic for best mineral levels; can soak or slow cook, otherwise oils oxidize when cooked.
Seeds	Add liberally to salads	As for nuts.
Tofu	Palm-sized piece up to twice a week, maximum	See soy info on page 68; choose good quality.
Garlic	One to two cloves, depending on your taste	Ideally organic fresh cloves, chopped or crushed. Can buy good-quality 'quick' garlic paste in tubes, jars or frozen.
Turmeric, cinnamon, paprika, curry powder, cumin, coriander	About one teaspoon total – more if you like	Buying ready ground is fine (organic where possible), unless you're used to grinding spices yourself. Change regularly – if a spice has lost its smell, it needs replacing.
Root ginger	Up to 12mm (½ inch), grated	Buy this in the vegetable section of the supermarket. Can also buy good-quality 'quick' ginger paste in tubes or chopped in jars, which can be a better alternative to the much less pungent ground spice, but check for sugar or additives.
Dried herbs, bay leaf	About half a teaspoon of dried herbs/one bay leaf	Buy in small quantities and replace often. Dried herbs are much less pungent than fresh, so you might use more.
Fresh herbs	A handful or more a day	Easiest to grow in pots in the kitchen or window sill; can be bought organically in good supermarkets to use liberally; they freeze well.

(continued)

Sources and quantities		
Ingredient	Amount per person	Healthy option
Creamed coconut	Half to whole 200g (7oz) block, grated or chopped fairly small	Buy organic blocks in health food shops or the healthy section of supermarkets. Chop off and add directly to dishes or make up milk by adding hot water: 200g (7oz) creamed coconut makes about 600ml (1 pint) of thickish coconut milk.
Lemons/ limes and their juice	Juice of one or two, to taste (see page 100 for adding to water)	Buy fresh as needed, but you can also keep dried lime slices in the cupboard for curries, or preserved lemons for Moroccan-type dishes. Bottles of lemon and/or lime juice are useful for cooking and to add to dressings and drinks.
Butter, coconut oil	For baking and cooking	These are saturated fats that are less damaging to body tissues when heated. Buy organic where possible and unsalted butter so you can add a little high-quality salt if needed – see below. If you want a spreadable butter, look for one with the least sunflower oil, so no 'low-fat' versions. Buy coconut oil from a health food shop, where it can be guaranteed not deodorized or hydrogenated.
Olive oil	For cooking and salads	Unrefined, cold-pressed, virgin – buy quality for higher anti-inflammatory oleocanthal and oleic acid; to absorb fat-soluble nutrients from salads.
Sea or rock salt	Sprinkle on food to taste	Can help tired adrenals when body low in sodium. Buy good quality, avoiding cheap table salt that is chemically processed and lacks the extra minerals in some rock salts – iron gives Himalayan salt its pink colour.

Health warning

Polyunsaturated oils like sunflower oil aren't recommended. Some cold-pressed versions of these, like sesame oil, can be used for dressings, but the refined types bought in plastic bottles provide too many omega-6 oils – and toxins from the plastic easily leach into the oil. Refined polyunsaturated oils should never be used for cooking as they are easily damaged by heat and produce harmful trans-fats.[7]

STEWS, CASSEROLES AND CURRIES

These can be eaten for lunch, dinner or even breakfast. You can leave them to slow cook all day for your evening meal, put them in a flask for lunch or freeze them in portion-sized packs for another day. Most benefit from long, slow cooking – especially if you're including beans or grains like buckwheat groats or pearl barley.

Here's how to make them:

Pick a flavouring

Choose from the following flavour 'families,' or create your own combos:

- Thai – chilli, coconut and lime with fresh ginger, or green Thai curry paste and lemon grass
- Mediterranean – garlic, basil, oregano, rosemary, thyme, bay leaves, optional chilli
- Indian – ginger, garlic, cumin, coriander, turmeric and chilli, or curry powder
- Moroccan – cinnamon, cumin, coriander, paprika, lemon
- Herby – garlic, parsley, thyme, chives, bay leaves

Choose some vegetables

According to season and availability; aim for a mixture of colours:

- Celery
- Cabbage or kale
- Broccoli or cauliflower
- Greens or pak choi
- Carrots
- Peppers
- Tomatoes
- Green beans
- Squash/pumpkin
- Parsnips
- Sweet potatoes
- Mushrooms
- Fennel
- Courgette

Add some protein

- Meat
- Fish
- Beans
- Lentils

- Chestnuts
- Cashew nuts
- Cheese
- Tofu

Cooking methods

Pan on the hob

1. Put some olive oil, butter or coconut oil in a pan. Add onions, garlic and flavourings, fry gently until they begin to soften.
2. Add the vegetables and stir them around for a few minutes until they begin to soften. Add the protein (or earlier if it takes longer to cook).
3. Add water or homemade, unsalted stock to cover all ingredients twice over. You can also add some woody herbs at this stage, like fresh thyme, rosemary and bay leaves.
4. Turn heat to lowest setting and cover pan; stir every so often to avoid sticking and burning. Cook for one to two hours for meat and raw pulses or 30–45 minutes for pre-cooked pulses, tofu or fish.

Electric slow cooker (crock-pot) – fast

1. Put all the ingredients in a pot and cover with twice as much water.
2. Cook for six hours on a medium heat or eight hours on a low heat.

Electric slow cooker with preparation

1. Follow the method above, but fry the flavourings and vegetables first, as in pan on the hob.
2. Before serving add seasonings like fresh chopped herbs, creamed coconut, lemon or lime juice, sea/rock salt and pepper, tamarind paste, yoghurt.

Health tip

Always use garlic and onions in abundance in your cooking if they suit you. They have been shown to be anti-inflammatory, immune-modulating and antibacterial, and they aid blood-sugar balance, circulation, detoxification and digestion.[8]

SALADS

A salad can be made up of any kind of raw and sometimes cooked vegetables, arranged together to form an attractive, colourful meal. Load up layers into a bowl, a soup plate or straight into a large lunch box. With dressing, a salad will last in the fridge for two consecutive meals, e.g. dinner and a packed lunch the next day.

Layer 1 – a handful of mixed green leaves

Spread these out to cover the bottom of the bowl/plate:

- Lettuce, especially the darker varieties like romaine or cos
- Watercress
- Rocket
- Baby spinach leaves (or larger leaves), or baby beet leaves 'cooked'*
- Herb leaf salad
- Mustard leaves

* With spinach or beet leaves there's the option to roughly chop them, put them in a colander in the sink, then pour over a kettle-full of boiling water to soften them up; allow to cool before adding to the bowl.

Layer 2 – vegetables

- Avocado
- Onion or spring onion, finely chopped
- Celery
- Mushrooms
- Peppers
- Tomatoes
- Cucumber
- Olives
- Roasted vegetables – warm or cold. Use those that keep their shape, like fennel, celery, red pepper, cherry tomatoes, whole garlic cloves, small onions, sweet potatoes roasted with some olive oil and optional rosemary
- A handful of any roughly chopped fresh herb leaf

Layer 3 – optional raw root vegetables

Serve these grated:

- Carrot
- Beetroot
- Celeriac
- Courgette

Layer 4 – protein

- Fish, meat or seafood – cold cuts, roasted meat or fish with olive oil and garlic, pan-fried slivers of liver, steak, duck, lamb, chicken or fish, still warm (my quick favourite: baked salmon fillet or chicken breast slathered in pesto)
- Cooked beans/pulses/lentils
- Handful of raw nuts or seeds like sunflower, pumpkin and sesame
- Hardboiled egg or omelette
- Goat's or feta cheese

Dressings and other tasty additions

- The easiest and quickest dressing is a splash of extra virgin olive oil and a smaller splash of cider vinegar, balsamic vinegar or lemon juice, straight onto the salad

- Olive oil, cider or wine vinegar, Dijon or wholegrain mustard and a tiny bit of good-quality honey, mixed together in a jar

- Tahini, an equal quantity of water, crushed garlic, juice of half a lemon (or more to taste) and a splash of soy sauce. Add a little bit of chilli too, if you like.

- A good-sized dollop of houmous or baba ghanoush

- Healthy sprinkles: lightly toasted or raw seeds, pine nuts or nuts, crispy onions, pickled or black garlic, capers, soaked seaweed, anchovies, fennel or cumin seeds, sprinkle of goat's cheese, a little rock or sea salt

STIR-FRIES

Stir-fries are the ultimate healthy convenience meal. Lower temperatures give you time to stir and check, with less chance of burning, and if you have a lid for your wok you can steam-fry, with a little water in the pan, giving you time to prepare other parts of the meal. You can miss out on the grain part, like rice or buckwheat noodles, entirely or have half a mug of grains and two to three portions of the vegetables per person as a good balance.

Group 1 vegetables

Cut these into equal sized batons/sticks:

- Carrots
- Celery
- Peppers

- Mushrooms
- Leeks
- Kohlrabi

Group 2 vegetables

Shred or chop these:

- Broccoli
- Kale
- Cabbage
- Chinese cabbage
- Pak choi

- Spring greens
- Spinach
- Chard
- Brussels sprouts
- Cavolo nero

Protein

- Tofu – cook this separately*
- Raw or cooked meat
- Prawns

- Firm white fish
- Cashew nuts
- Roasted almonds

*To cook the tofu, cut it into cubes and fry in a shallow layer of coconut oil until lightly brown on all sides. Then tip into a bowl containing a mixture of soy sauce (or gluten-free tamari), finely grated ginger, crushed garlic and optional chilli. Stir it around, then return to the pan and stir and fry until dry and sticky.

You can give the meat and fish the same kind of treatment, and experiment with the flavourings; this works particularly well with leftover lamb or duck.

Cooking method

Melt one to two tablespoons of coconut oil in a wok, deep frying pan or a large saucepan. Add one chopped medium onion per person, stir and fry for two or three minutes. Add crushed garlic and grated fresh ginger – at least one dessertspoon.

1. Add group 1 vegetables and stir-fry for a couple of minutes. Put the lid on if you have one, otherwise continue stirring and frying for about five minutes, until the vegetables begin to soften. Finely sliced raw meat can go in at this stage – stir and fry until nearly cooked.

2. Add green leaves, along with softer proteins like fish, prawns and cooked meats. Continue to stir and fry for a few minutes until the greens just begin to wilt and the meat or fish is cooked.

3. Add the tofu, cashew nuts or the separately cooked meat at this stage and sprinkle with fresh, chopped coriander.

COOKING WITH GRAINS AND BEANS

Eat grains and beans with foods rich in vitamin A and carotenoids (fat-soluble nutrients) found in meat, butter and deep-coloured vegetables, especially orange roots and dark green leaves, for best iron absorption.[9]

Reduce phytic acid and lectins

Soak beans overnight, change the water in the morning and leave to soak again during the day. Change the water again and then cook for one to two hours depending on the type and age of the bean. If you do large batches you can freeze portion-sized bags once they've cooled, and you'll have a ready supply to use in salads or cooking, without the toxic metals present in tins. You don't have to defrost them before use if cooking.

Cook with vegetables

Cooking grains and beans with vegetables has been shown to help reduce their phytic acid content, especially when slow-cooked to break it down further.[10] Grains and beans are traditionally cooked with garlic and onion to make iron and zinc more available.[11] Other members of this family – shallots, spring onions, leeks, and chives – will also work, as well as providing insulin-regulating, circulation-supporting sulphur compounds.

Use acidifiers

These are flavourings added to cooking that also break down anti-nutrients. They include amchur (or amchoor, mango powder), lime powder, tamarind, fruit, dried fruit, fruit juice – all of which can be added to soaking or cooking – and yoghurt, for a lactic acid pre-soak.

If you're a vegan

You need to take more care to soak beans for at least 24 hours (changing the water at least once or twice) before cooking with an acidifier and eating alongside foods high in vitamin C (e.g. lots of coloured veg in a side salad) to help iron absorption. These can be pre-cooked and frozen in portions. Heat-cooking grains and beans has been shown to increase iron bioavailability but to decrease that of zinc[12] – commonly low in vegans.

BEST STARCHY CHOICES

Depending on your tastes and energy needs, you may wish to add a small portion of grains to your breakfast or lunch. Try and minimize wheat to reduce the gluten in your diet, and vary the types you choose from the list below so you don't subject your immune system to the same lectins over and over again.[13] The following are all gluten-free:

- Quinoa and wild rice – the most alkalizing grains

- Basmati brown rice – best for blood sugar but extremely high in phytic acid, so eat just two to three times a week

- Millet and buckwheat – these cause the fewest immune reactions

- Buckwheat groats – great in stews

- Sweet potatoes – less starchy than white potatoes

- New potatoes – with skins intact, these are the best potato choice; have baked potatoes as an occasional lunch treat only

You'll find meal plans and more recipes at www.charlottewattshealth.com

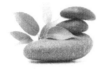

CHAPTER 11

A Morning Revolution

'Whatever you can do, or dream you can, begin it.
Boldness has genius, power and magic in it.'
JOHANN WOLFGANG VON GOETHE

One of the most profound things you can do for your health is to start your day well. What you do in the morning vastly influences your food choices, energy levels and ability to cope with life's challenges throughout the day. This means better-quality sleep and, therefore, waking refreshed the next day.

The common twenty-first-century routine of jangly alarm, shoot out of bed, check smartphone, rush breakfast and ping out the door (not naked, there's hurried dressing in there too) is obviously a recipe for a stress hormone-charged start. That plays round again, with a stressy day feeding poor-quality sleep, and you know the rest... If getting up earlier for all this good stuff seems too demanding right now, allowing even a bit of extra time will soon feed into waking more refreshed.

STRONG FOUNDATIONS TO BUILD GOOD CHOICES

By waking smoothly and taking just a bit of time to prepare yourself for the day's demands, you can give yourself space to taste and enjoy food that's good for digestion and appetite regulation; sustaining food rescues you from frustrating and exhausting daytime highs and lows. A good breakfast time is our most important tool for breaking the stress loops we explored in chapter 5.

Breakfast is the meal that can either set up your good mood, energy and coping capacity for the coming day or set you off on a giddy ride of bouncing between craving quick fixes and struggling for motivation. The right meal after the long period without food overnight can have the greatest knock-on effect on your food choices throughout the day. Those 4 p.m. and late-night sweet or crisp cravings can be traced back to the wrong input at the start of your day, when a nasty game of energy 'catch-up' can have you in the grip of cravings and mood swings all day.

You probably already know how a good breakfast makes sense, but until you've experienced the effects it can have, the habit won't stick. As we learned earlier, habits are created out of rich 'sense memories' based on experienced senses and feelings, so you won't truly create a real paradigm shift, a new way of living, without finding a nourishing and satisfying morning routine that works for you.

The most important meal of the day

Skipping breakfast has been shown to cause weight, focus, mood and appetite problems.[1,2] Our metabolism is designed to take in most calories in the first half of each day to fuel the search for more food. A protein-rich breakfast, in particular, has been shown to satisfy appetite for longer than a high-carb breakfast (like cereal),[3] and healthy fats (see page 100) included at breakfast show better results in the level of morning blood-sugar balance than low-fat options.[4]

Many people who struggle to lose weight eat little for breakfast and lunch and pile up the calories – often as refined carbs – towards the end of the day, when digestion and metabolism have slowed, making excess more likely to be laid down as fat. Skipping breakfast in an attempt to lose weight will backfire,[5] as it tends to result in poor food choices throughout the day and even overeating later. If you don't fuel up on rising, stress hormones take over to raise blood-sugar levels, which means you're starting the day from a fear-based state.

Think outside the (cereal) box

Our morning routines are yet another casualty of our over-subscribed diaries, leaving breakfast less of a meal – with variety and enjoyment – and more a glorified convenience snack. Many people feel they are at least eating healthily at this meal, but tea and toast or boxed cereals are really just comfort foods.

Look at eating habits across the world and you'll notice that the foods we consider breakfast fare in the West come from a fairly small range of choices. People eat grilled fish and vegetables for breakfast in Korea, fish and coconut *sambol* in Sri Lanka, dim sum in some parts of Thailand, and meats, smoked fish and cheeses in Scandinavian countries – choices that are more nutritionally supportive than the glut of processed grain products such as cereals and breads most of us eat. It's no coincidence that the typical Western breakfast of boxed cereal, white bread and high-sugar jam has soared in popularity alongside the rise of obesity, diabetes and heart disease.

The bottom-line breakfast rule is simple: *eat healthy food you enjoy*. You can eat anything at breakfast, even last night's leftover curry (my favourite). All of the lunch and dinner suggestions in the previous and coming chapters make great breakfasts too, and are an easy way to prepare food in advance. Stew is a great on a cold winter's day.

Wake-up call

For the die-hard 'don't eat until 11 a.m.' types, consider this period of waking up your morning metabolism your new project for weeks 1–3 of De-Stress Eating and wean yourself slowly. Even just the smoothie on page 166 or some nuts is a good start.

Start the day with the juice of half a lemon in hot water to wake up your liver and digestion in a clean, healthy way. Drink this about 20 minutes before breakfast – you can also add slices of fresh ginger to warm up or calm the digestion, and/or cinnamon to sweeten and improve blood-sugar balance.

If you're used to having a cup of coffee or tea before breakfast, save this until you have food in your stomach. If you drink coffee or tea when blood-sugar levels are low, you'll get a surge as your body produces adrenaline in response to the caffeine and you won't feel the need for food to raise them.

The De-Stress breakfast		
What	Why	How
Protein	Shown to satisfy appetite for longer, raise metabolism, keep insulin production low and reduce fat-storing tendencies.	Animal proteins like meat, fish, eggs or dairy provide complete protein – all the amino acid building blocks we need to help build muscle. Eating eggs for breakfast has been shown to help weight loss[6] as they improve glucose/insulin response and food choices for the rest of the day.[7,8] Keep nut butters like hazelnut and pumpkin seed in the fridge for a quick protein and healthy fat addition to rye bread or crackers. For vegans, including beans and pulses in breakfast can provide important protein to help cope with the day's stress; try the stews on page 123.
Complex carbs	Not only starches like bread and cereal. The best brain and muscle fuel also comes from other complex carbohydrate in whole plant sources such as nuts, seeds, fruit and vegetables.[9]	Best-case scenario is using breakfast as another opportunity for a vegetable portion: avocados, watercress, tomatoes and spinach all make perfect breakfast foods. Fruit is best as an energy source when kept intact, and not with fibre removed as a juice, so eat your fruit whole. Add energy from nuts to porridge or cereal soaked overnight for digestibility.

Use the De-Stress Energy and Mood Monitoring Chart at www.charlottewattshealth.com to compare how different breakfast combinations make you feel in terms of cravings, 'highs and lows' and appetite.

Here are three breakfast options to try:

1. Breakfast outside the box

This is the best basis for starting the day, especially if you tend towards sugar cravings; it can be prepared the night before as you make dinner:

Choose a protein source

- Eggs: one or two boiled, poached, slowly scrambled or omelette
- Fish: smoked mackerel, trout or salmon fillet
- Goat's or sheep's cheese – i.e. feta or soft cheese
- Two slices of turkey or chicken
- (Occasionally) good-quality ham or bacon, Parma ham (usually prepared without nitrates)
- Portion of prepared beans, falafel or nut burger if vegan

Choose vegetables

Add a palm-sized portion of at least two of the following (or any other veg):

- Avocado
- Tomatoes
- Asparagus
- Spinach
- Watercress
- Cucumber
- Cooked beetroot (not in vinegar)
- Rocket
- Artichokes

2. The healthy 'British'

This is a good 'grounding' breakfast for the recovering sugar junkie:

- Eggs: poached, slowly scrambled or omelette
- Good-quality free-range bacon (two slices) or sausage (one or two, depending on size), grilled – just once or twice a week total, as they contain nitrate preservatives (unless you can buy them without). Alternatively, a high-quality lamb or beef burger is a nitrate-free occasional option. For a vegetarian or different protein option, either grill two Portobello mushrooms (with olive oil), halloumi or good-quality nut burgers.

- Two halves of a medium tomato, grilled, or four to six cherry tomatoes oven roasted with a little olive oil

- Optional vegetable portion: wilted spinach or asparagus

- Add a third of a can of baked beans – choose low sugar or a brand sweetened with apple juice, such as Whole Earth

If you find you're better suited to a small portion of starchy carb with your savoury breakfast, buy more expensive, quality breads. Loaves can be sliced and frozen and then individual portions pulled out to make toast. Sourdough rye is better digested and evidence indicates that rye bread may boost feelings of fullness when eaten at breakfast.[10] Eat with butter, nut butters or olive oil – no hydrogenated or high-sunflower oil spreads.

3. Bircher muesli medley

This is the best alternative to regular muesli if you want a morning starchy carb; the oats and nuts are soaked and so are easier to digest and lower in phytic acid:

1. Soak 35g (about two tablespoons) of rolled oats in yoghurt – or alternatively, water or half-water/half-freshly squeezed apple juice – overnight in the fridge with a tablespoon of nuts and seeds for protein: choose from almonds, Brazils, walnuts, pecans, sunflower and pumpkin seeds. You can add a dessertspoon of golden linseeds for increased detoxifying, digestive and hormonal health.

2. Sweeten only with ground cinnamon, unsweetened desiccated coconut and fruit from the following options: chopped dried apricots, prunes, grated apple, berries, sliced or stewed plums and/or apples, unsweetened purees.

3. For variety, or a gluten-free option, buckwheat, quinoa or millet flakes can be used in place of oats or mixed in with them.

4. You can add a dollop of plain live Greek or whole milk yoghurt to taste if using oats soaked in water/apple juice.

5. For speed, mix up your grains, nuts and seeds and keep in an airtight container to pour quickly into a bowl.

GOOD MORNING!

Nourishing yourself isn't only about what you eat, but *how* you eat it. Here's the ideal De-Stress morning routine, with options depending on the amount of time you have. Taking any of the attitudes on board is a positive move and will impact on your stress levels and mood throughout the day.

1. Wake up and give yourself time (even 30 seconds) before leaping into action; take a few deep breaths to increase oxygen flow through your brain and even prepare a positive outlook for the day with the gratitude practice on page 161.

2. Ease out of bed by sitting on the side and then standing up slowly. This tells your body there's no imminent danger. Have a stretch to wake up your muscles and nervous system and try some of the movements on pages 209–12 to invite connective tissues to loosen. Rub and tap your body, move hands, feet and neck as feels natural to promote the body awareness that can prevent you from just living neck-up for the rest of the day.

3. Avoid looking at any tech or incoming information that distracts you away from the present towards thinking or reacting modes until at least an hour after waking – until you start the working day during the week, and a whole morning at weekends if possible. If your brain tends to be agitated on waking, writing down an unedited stream of consciousness in a diary or notebook can download the chatter.

4. Drink some lemon juice with hot water and optional cinnamon and ginger.

5. Consider a walk, meditation, breathing exercise or morning yoga sequence: movement is best before food so digestion doesn't steal energy from your muscles. Set a soft alarm for the time allotted so no

panic sets in. Don't feel you have to spend the same amount of time every morning and if you miss one session, just start again the next day. Your differing routines will set the pace; be sure to finish before low morning blood-sugar levels make you feel woozy.

6. Make breakfast. Stick to the task and feel like this is an important part of self-care. Prepare some things the night before, to make the process as simple as possible. Don't just start bolting your food while standing up or take it with you while you get ready; sit at a table and place it in front of you, then take 10 deep breaths to prepare for digestion.

7. Eat breakfast. Eat calmly and take at least 15 minutes, chewing every mouthful and actually tasting your food. If you eat slowly enough and chew well, you should naturally allow digestion to happen more easily. Include sitting for five minutes after you've finished eating as part of your breakfast time. If you usually watch TV at breakfast, switch to listening to the radio to reduce screen time.

8. Enjoy what you eat. If you didn't, make changes the next day, but if you're missing a sweeter breakfast, it can take a few days for your taste buds to change.

9. Ease into your day. If you're not taking time for breathing, meditation and so on after breakfast, you may want to jump into action after eating, but anything you can do to support a calm state can help your food go down, ensure full digestion and keep you sated until lunchtime.

10. If travelling, use the time as space for yourself. If on a train or bus, avoid dropping into emails or social networking and watch the world go by, read a book, listen to calming music, an audio meditation or audiobook. If driving, find a calming radio station or drive and breathe mindfully, being with your reactions if the traffic gets bad!

Are you taking second place to the family?

If you're bolting your food down between feeding the kids, dog and husband, watch where this is being put upon you and where you're letting it happen. Remember, if you don't make even a little space for yourself (just 10 breaths?), you'll eventually run out of energy to look after other people and let stress-inducing resentment build in the process. Find days when you're looked after – or even have the kids looked after. Just once a week or every fortnight can make a difference. Eat with the kids to encourage them to be more mindful and therefore create space for you; they can eat the same food as you, or versions of it.

Those stressy habits resolved

*   If waking is difficult see the sleep solutions on pages 160–61. You may want to do a simple breathing exercise or mindfulness practice before getting out of bed.

*   If you're used to running out of the door as soon as you've stuffed in breakfast, it can really reclaim the day to take a pause before you go.

*   If you have only 2–10 minutes for an exercise routine, try the movements on pages 209–12.

*   Take a stroll around the block or a short run if you're an exercise bunny, but not to the point of feeling adrenaline kicking in – this is individual but you'll know it by your heart suddenly racing.

*   If you leave for work, leave with a smile. If you work from home, separate your working environment from your morning preparation; even go for a walk around the block as if you're 'going to work'. If it's a weekend, factor in time on at least one day to rest for an hour or two after breakfast to decompress properly from the week.

Troubleshooting

Problem: You get the 6:30 a.m. train or have a long drive to work and then eat breakfast at your desk.

Solution: Prioritize breakfast before work or pack a smoothie containing coconut milk and berries. If you have your breakfast on the train or at your desk, focus on eating it, with no work or phone calls at the same time. Try soup, stew or porridge in a flask during the colder months. Keep nut butters at work to add to sourdough rye or crackers, try the suggested snack bars on page 168 and nuts for days when you have less time.

Problem: You go to the gym before work and never know what to eat.

Solution: This routine can mean not eating for a few hours after getting up – not a good idea with intense exercise in which levels of stress hormones are raised. Have a smoothie with coconut milk and berries beforehand to provide energy and then eat your full breakfast straight after for protein to replenish muscle.

Help for your specific Stress Suit		
	You may find that you...	Best single change you could make
Stressed and Wired	start the day in a frenzy of stress hormones	Make time to do a full 15-minute calming activity to retrain your nervous system.
Stressed and Tired	drag yourself to vertical and really don't want to get out of bed	Have a protein breakfast and chew thoroughly; make at least a little time to build up energy through full breathing.
Stressed and Cold	feel sluggish and heavy as you haul yourself upright	Get moving slowly and stretch to get your circulation going; include ginger in your morning hot lemon.
Stressed and Bloated	feel uncomfortable first thing and have an unsatisfactory bowel movement or none	Have hot lemon in water to stimulate liver and pancreas function; eat calmly and chew!

(continued)

Help for your specific Stress Suit		
	You may find that you...	Best single change you could make
Stressed and Sore	wake feeling heady, itchy or phlegmy	Choose the activity that most calms you to stop setting off these inflammatory reactions.
Stressed and Demotivated	feel no joy or downright dread for the coming day	Choose a meditation or breathing exercise that works for you to do sitting up in bed. Ensure protein for brain chemistry.
Stressed and Hormonal	wake feeling irritable and tetchy	Include liver-supporting foods for breakfast, such as smoked salmon or mackerel, nuts, seeds, avocado, beetroot and watercress.

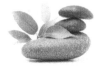

CHAPTER 12

Recharging Daytime

*'When people you greatly admire appear to be thinking
deep thoughts, they probably are thinking about lunch.'*
DOUGLAS ADAMS

This chapter focuses on daytime eating and living in the working week, or
when demands on time are high. Get this right and you can reclaim time
from weekends and holidays when you may have been simply recovering
from the previous stress-load.

RECHARGING IS AN IMPORTANT PART OF WORK

If you're wondering why so many of us feel exhausted by 4 p.m. during
the week, here's food for thought: seven out of 10 office workers don't
leave their desks at lunchtime and a staggering 7 million Brits skip their
lunch breaks altogether.[1] For some, this is an attempt to get through a
pile of work or to get home earlier, but the truth is, failing to take time to
recharge is known to affect productivity and creativity and increases the
likelihood of making mistakes that steal time later.

If you're a parent, the same applies – and you may feel even more
pressure to put your needs further down the list. But any mode of
ploughing through without space made for regrouping and grounding
doesn't help our mood, social skills or reflective decision-making. Breaks

really are needed to keep our stress levels manageable and to feel we're being true to our best abilities. We all know that getting grumpy with our colleagues or children creates ripples that feed into stress loops.

During the course of the average high-pressure day, demands are put on our bodies in terms of functioning, maintenance and recovery. That means the essential nutrients we need to cope with the mental stress we're under – B vitamins, vitamin C, magnesium and zinc, to name a few – are quickly used up by the body's stress response. Unless we choose meals that replenish these nutrients and provide slow-feed energy, we can soon find ourselves caught in the roller-coaster loops that send us towards coffee, chocolate and crisps.

A decent lunch isn't just about what you eat, but how you set the scene for the chance to refuel intelligently; for full digestion, recovery time to 'just be' and acknowledgement that serving your needs in this way is at least as important as ticking off the to-do list.

Make your own lunch

Eating food you've prepared yourself, even a few days a week, promotes the feeling of self-care, connection and making the healthiest choices you can. Plus, cooking more dinners at home means more healthy leftovers for lunch the next day.

Make about 30 per cent of your lunch protein (see page 98); it takes longer to digest and will keep you well fuelled and feeling fuller for longer, but take time to chew! If you're eating meat and can't afford or find organic varieties, read the labels to ensure you're buying wild or free-range options to which no sugars, salts, processed fats or preservatives such as sodium or potassium nitrate have been added (Parma ham is usually okay).

Omelettes or frittatas made with plenty of vegetables (and feta cheese) and eaten with a huge raw salad make for a great protein-rich lunch and will last a few meals. Vegetables and salad should make up the bulk of your lunch, especially green leafy vegetables where you can. A salad of avocado, fresh herb leaves, greens such as watercress, rocket or chicory and lots of brightly coloured vegetables such as grated beetroot, carrots and courgettes, sliced tomatoes, cucumber, celery and peppers should accompany your protein choice at least four times a week. Sprinkle on seeds and add olive oil for brain-satisfying fats.

Stews are a great way of getting your vegetable nutrients and to hydrate naturally (see Chapter 10). You can prepare them beforehand (Sunday is good) and freeze them in containers; take into work in a large thermos or heat up at lunchtime.

Lunchtime do's and don'ts

Do:

- Use lunch to increase your vegetable intake. Having vegetables only at dinner won't provide enough of the fibre, vitamins and minerals a productive body needs.

- Experiment during your six-week plan with a portion of either grains or beans at lunch. Some people find that grains actually increase their appetite and make them sleepy, so if this is you, choose only protein and vegetables at lunch. Use the troubleshooters on page 113.

- If you're buying out and really want a sandwich, look for shops that sell alternatives to wheat bread, such as rye, and avoid malted breads, as the brown colour comes from added *maltose*, a form of sugar. Sourdough bread, in which the problematic gluten is more broken down, is now more widely available.

Don't:

- Have a sandwich every day. If you do eat bread, have several days off gluten-containing wheat or rye each week by choosing a hearty soup or salad as an alternative.

- Choose refined carbohydrates. White bread, pastries and pies release energy too quickly and provide 'empty' calories that quickly turn to fat. Wouldn't dream of eating cake for lunch? Having such refined carbohydrates is, in nutritional terms, very similar.

At-work lunch store cupboard

The following items can be kept in a drawer ready for when you can buy a few fresh bits on the way to work:

- Extra virgin olive oil

- Balsamic vinegar or lemon juice

- Tins of salmon, sardines and mackerel

- Packs of pre-cooked beans like lentils or aduki beans

- Sealed tubs of almonds, cashews, sunflower and pumpkin seeds

You can then make up a salad any time from bags of watercress or rocket, avocados, other salad veg, fresh protein like smoked salmon or Parma ham and optional houmous.

How you have lunch

Nourishing yourself isn't only about *what* you eat, but *how* you eat it. Explore options so you can vary them depending on how much time you have. Here's how to have a stress-free lunchtime:

- If you can choose your lunch time, when you begin to feel hungry, go and prepare or buy your lunch. Take 10 deep breaths before eating it, to punctuate the end of the morning and calm any leftover stress response that could hinder your digestion.

- Try and resist the urge to nip to the nearest take-away; instead stroll to somewhere you know there is better choice.

- Having lunch in a park with a friend ticks many De-Stress boxes. If you can't manage this, a café or staff room is better than a desk for a social/rest/quick fix with real people rather than a computer screen.

- Allow 15 minutes after eating for digestion and then take a walk. If you are of a more introverted nature, you may well need the whole break to have some peace alone, to recharge away from the herd and the noise.

- If you like your coffee, have it after lunch. This will help slow down the rate at which coffee releases adrenaline into your system and prevent you feeling stress later in the afternoon. Swap a milky latte for an Americano with a little hot milk.

- If you go to the gym at lunchtime, have an easily digested snack beforehand and then lunch straight afterwards.

Post-lunch bloating?

Creating a habit of taking 10 deep breaths before eating relaxes your body to prepare it for receiving food and minimizing stress-related gassiness or bloating. Try and avoid wheat-containing sandwiches, pizza, noodles, pasta and quiche. Add dried spices such as star anise, fennel and ginger and fresh herbs to your lunch to aid digestion and reduce gas. Choose potassium-rich vegetables such as cucumber, parsley and asparagus for a diuretic effect that can prevent the fluid build-up that stress hormones can create. Simple home-made organic chicken and vegetable stews can be most healing for a stressed gut.

Get some light

A 10-minute walk to a nearby park or café can ensure you get a mood-enhancing vitamin D and serotonin hit, especially in the winter when you may not see any daylight during the morning or evening hours. Low levels of serotonin can prompt the urge for sugar to raise levels in the brain – common during the dark winter months. If it's a dull day, try to be outside at lunchtime for half an hour or more, finding oxygenating greenery if you can. If it's sunny, 10 minutes can top you up.

Transform your lunchtime routine into a more supportive one		
Stressy lunch	Finding your balance	De-Stress success
Ready meal	Allow a few of these each week, if needs be, and do a little research into the healthiest and most easily available for those difficult times.	Look for high-protein soups containing, for example, pea and ham, chicken and hearty lentils – to help keep you going. If you must have a ready meal, check labels for ingredients you simply don't recognize as food. Indian and spicy dishes often have fewer preservatives as the spices themselves preserve food well.
A bought-in salad that never satisfies	Ensure a salad is high enough in protein and good fat to satisfy you for the rest of the afternoon. Add avocado and seeds if needed. A 'gloopy' pasta or potato 'salad' choice is never a good option.	Look for a salad that contains a palm-sized protein portion (about 100–150g (3½–5oz) and good fats in the form of any one or two of the following: avocado, olives, rapeseed, olive or sesame oil, a few mixed nuts or seeds. Check dressing labels for sugar content – a ready-made salad dressing labelled 'low fat' may be high in sugar.
Client lunches with good wine on offer	If you feel that saying 'no' to alcohol isn't an option, have a couple of glasses of water beforehand, so you don't arrive thirsty and drink wine to get hydrated (doesn't work). Add some sparkling mineral water or a few ice cubes to your wine to dilute it.	Dense protein (egg, fish, meat) and plenty of veg will help your liver handle alcohol. Remember, you don't have to justify not drinking at lunchtime (or at any other time, for that matter!), but peer group pressure really is unacceptable.

INTO THE AFTERNOON

There are many alternatives to the food pick-me-ups and distractions (like Facebook) we often turn to when flagging. These help you move with, rather than push against, your natural energy flows:

- If you feel your mind dropping into a 'dull' phase, learn to just go with it and try the essential mindful practice of patience and taking breaks. Our brains move through the same cycles of varying brainwave frequencies awake as when we're asleep, we just experience them consciously.

- Your brain regulates the amount of information it receives to protect itself from overload. When it needs some crucial downtime, you can find yourself day-dreaming or in the same alpha-wave meditative state where you may have been staring out of the window and suddenly noticed that 10 minutes have passed. Go with it and resist the urge to crank up with caffeine; we can panic that we're too tired to get what we need done, but if you allow a mind-rest, you'll be able to feel the pick-up into a refreshed state, where a new perspective on an old problem may be waiting.

- If you feel frustration or blockage with the work you're doing, switch modes to find something that needs a different mental skillset. So if you're writing, do something practical like filing or tidying (this book is sponsored by the washing-up!), or if trying to analyse, find something creative like a design job… or just doodle. Cortisol dampens the hippocampus, the part of the brain where we form new memories, and this is shown to shrink with sustained stress; shifting gears to de-stress helps you to retain facts you need for efficiency.

- Visualizing light is a traditional technique to 'brighten the mind'. It can be done any time of day, whenever it's needed, and floods the brain with a surge of noradrenaline, the neurotransmitter that creates clarity and alertness.

- Rub the roof of your mouth with the tip of your tongue – you can feel the tickling sensation waking up your brain by stimulating nerves directly into it.

- Be aware of your posture and sit up straight whenever you notice you're slumping (see page 187 for why). Lift up through the back of the skull to counter the 'chin lifting' common when we hunch and then look up at screens. Opening the chest and tucking the chin lightly towards your throat allows stress to drain down from your neck and shoulders. Stand up and stretch whenever you need to.

Clever napping

A nap of 15–30 minutes mid-afternoon lets your brain do some vital housekeeping. While the logical left side relaxes, the right side clears out temporary storage areas, pushes information into long-term storage and solidifies your memories from the day.[2] This relieves stress when we struggle to remember things and prevents us from relying on stress hormones or stimulants when getting enough sleep eludes us.

Any longer, though, and moving into deeper sleep cycles can result in grogginess rather than rejuvenation and interfere with sleep quality overnight. This is individual: naps suit some people – those able to drop down and then up out of deep sleep quickly. If not, a snooze can leave a feeling of being 'wiped out'.

Help for your specific Stress Suit		
	You may find that you...	Best single change you could make
Stressed and Wired	are far too busy to stop for lunch	Adding just five to 10 minutes to your break can make a difference. If you're really pushed for time, have a hearty soup that's easier to digest.
Stressed and Tired	feel an energy slump after lunch	See the caffeine section on page 172. Try liquorice tea for natural energy production.
Stressed and Cold	feel tired from the morning's activities	Make sure you get some cold or fresh air, particularly if your office is stuffy.
Stressed and Bloated	bloat or feel discomfort after eating lunch	Follow your lunch with dandelion, mint, fennel or nettle tea.
Stressed and Sore	can feel stress-related inflammatory symptoms after lunch	Keep a food diary to monitor which types of lunch affect you.
Stressed and Demotivated	feel you might need to console yourself with 'bad' foods	Phone a trusted friend who makes you laugh instead, or pick a breathing exercise that makes you feel centred.
Stressed and Hormonal	just want sweet foods before and around the time of your period	If you need to succumb, be very clear about choosing quality treats and then enjoy them only after a healthy lunch.

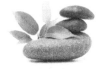

CHAPTER 13

Mindful Evenings

'All the tragedy in the world, in the individual and in the multitude, comes from lack of harmony. And harmony is best given by producing harmony in one's life.'
HAZRAT INAYAT KHAN

Just as what you do and eat in the morning sets the tone for how you'll feel and function throughout the day, so your evening routine sets the tone for the next morning. Yet we often fight our natural impulse towards a relaxing, sleep-inducing evening, believing we might be missing out if we're not having an extremely exciting time.

In the modern world this often means drinking alcohol if out with friends or TV overload if staying in. Looking at how these activities affect our sleep can help us find a balance between enjoyment, health and weight loss.

Evening is the time when cortisol levels are lowering to reduce stimulation and prepare the body for rest. Stress taken into the evening can not only keep you awake, it can increase the likelihood of your body laying down fat.[1] Evening relaxation of both body and brain helps keep your appetite appropriate for the low level of activity that your body expects at night, and helps your digestion at a time when it's slowing down.

Your brain is only around 3 per cent of your body weight but it uses around 20 per cent of your energy and up to 70 per cent when you're stressed. It needs to slow down – not just to get to sleep, but to drop into the deeper sleep cycles it needs in order to dream and process the day's input.

The hours when you're unconscious are some of the most important in your life.[2] In order for you to function fully while awake, your body relies on the immune-modulation, detoxification, tissue- and muscle-healing and mental-sorting processes that occur during this time.[3] If you don't respect this, chances are you'll experience fatigue, irritability, poor concentration, weight gain and poor recovery from stress, injury and skin complaints.

TIRED, BUT NOT SLEEPY

Chronic tiredness at night is common, and often about physical difficulties dealing with stress. After days of commuting, looking after children, working eight–18 hours with no lunch break and evenings spent texting or surfing the net, it's reasonable to feel tired. Our body clocks – that is, the 24-hour daily metabolic rhythms set into our biochemistry – have been set from when we lived in caves.[4] They follow the light-dark cycles of the sun, but continue even when we don't see daylight.[5]

This means ideally waking at sunrise and going to bed at sunset, obviously not something your average twenty-first-century dweller is doing. Simply putting lights on when it's dark outside, watching TV and surfing the net disrupt this system, which is naturally designed to shut you down for rest and recovery.[6] Our ancestors would have wound down by socializing with the tribe, chatting, eating, dancing and having sex – all heartily recommended De-Stress evening activities.

Sleep supporters

Try the following for at least half of your week, or have a monthly 'holiday at home' with the activities below each night for a week. This is great for stressful times when your sleep has become affected and you've slipped into those over-stimulating evening habits:

- Evaluate where your social life might be draining rather than recharging you. Does one night out make you feel connected and happy, whereas two in a row leave you having difficulty falling asleep and prone to craving refined carbs the next day?

- See the alcohol section on page 175 to reflect on going out without regrets.

- Communicate only with people who make you feel comforted and safe, not whipping up difficult emotional issues at a time when you need your brain to relax. This includes phone conversations, discerning social media and real physical interaction.

- Avoid all stimulants past 4 p.m. – caffeine, alcohol, sugar and even the TV or computer once you're home from work.

- If you need a stress release, put on your favourite music and dance and sing to your heart's content.

- Have a 'tech amnesty' at least an hour before bed, as flashing images and light close to the face from laptops and phone screens affect melatonin production, which can make it harder to get to sleep.

- Letting yourself 'be bored' and not turning automatically to habitual distractions of email and social media can stimulate creative hobbies instead. Go *old skool* and reconnect with things you used to enjoy, like drawing, sewing, playing a musical instrument, crosswords and – my favourite – jigsaws!

- Anything you do at the end of the day should be moving you towards a calm 'alpha' brain state: baths, reading non-thrilling books, listening to soothing music, a calm yoga practice or meditation will ensure quality rest.

- Don't fight it if you're tired: go to bed early and allow yourself to catch up on sleep.

- Aim to have as consistent as possible a bedtime and wake time, to let your body feel safe in its rhythm. Aim to be in bed by 10–11 p.m. as often as possible; the hours before midnight can be more restorative than those after, and staying up past then prompts cortisol release to keep you awake.

- Keep TVs, tablets and computers from your bedroom as much as possible. Maintain it as a haven for relaxation; don't work there, and keep lighting low.

- Sleep in a chilly and fully dark room. Too much heat or light (even on skin) can halt the production of melatonin; use blackout curtains if needed.

- Remove as many electrical devices from your bedroom as you can. Electro-Magnetic Fields (EMFs) from TVs and phone chargers can disrupt your sleep quality. Switch off your wi-fi at night and use an alarm clock rather than your phone by your bed.

Evening exercise

For many, evening is the only time they can find to exercise, but leave it too late and the nervous system excitation this can cause can affect sleep neurotransmitters. Our best cardiovascular efficiency and muscle strength is around 5 p.m., so straight after work is a great time to exercise and is best for the heart. Exercising outdoors helps to keep you connected to the natural world in terms of daylight and temperature, whereas more bright lights might artificially tell your body that it's another time of day entirely.

If evening is your chosen time, end with something that actively calms your nervous system. Yoga has been shown to help people sleep better and longer[7,8] and even just one restorative yoga posture (see Evening Practice from page 228) or 10 minutes of focused breathing can calm you down for a restful night's sleep.

See page 147 for nutritional guidelines around exercise.

Evening food

Living in the twenty-first century means we're far removed from the 5 p.m. 'tea time' that was a staple a generation or two ago. Now, many of us may not get home until 8 p.m., when the last thing we feel like doing is spending hours cooking our evening meal. This can leave us at the mercy of ready meals and eating later than our bodies want for digestion. Prioritizing breakfast and lunch as larger meals helps accommodate your energy and nutrient needs throughout the day, so you don't get home as famished and feel better equipped to make healthier choices in the evening.

After weeks 1–3 of the De-Stress Eating plan, your body should begin to get used to being fed better during the day. Without a string of blood-sugar highs and lows, you may become less inclined to overeat at night and your body has a chance to regenerate and rebuild itself during sleep rather than working overtime to digest an oversized evening meal. If you need carbs for refuelling after exercise, or tend to binge late at night, choose 'high-satiety' foods that don't upset body chemistry: a small portion of new potatoes in their skins is almost three times as satisfying as pasta, chips or rice and can stave off sweet cravings after a meal.[9]

You may go through a few days when your evening meal doesn't seem filling enough, but this will help to wake up morning hunger so you want a more satisfying breakfast – crucial if you've been skipping it. This chapter will show you how to make the right choices to help your brain generate its own essential neurotransmitters, or 'happy chemicals', such as dopamine, melatonin and serotonin, which it needs for sound sleep and mood stabilization, especially during times of chronic stress.

Brain sleep foods

Optimizing serotonin and other inhibitory or calming neurotransmitters also helps levels of GABA, the calming chemical that helps us switch off[10] and supports immunity.[11] It's known as our brain's 'natural braking system' and low levels are associated with anxiety and panic attacks as well as insomnia. Supplements for sleep are recommended in the free De-Stress Supplement Guide at www.charlottewattshealth.com – to help you produce GABA and serotonin naturally; in particular magnesium, vitamin B6 and taurine are recommended.

Glutamine-rich De-Stress foods, which help produce GABA, include bananas, broccoli, citrus fruits, halibut, lentils, nuts and organ meats. Tryptophan-rich De-Stress foods, which help produce serotonin, include almonds, avocados, bananas, beetroot, chicken, cottage cheese, duck, figs, mackerel, pheasant, salmon, sunflower seeds, tofu and turkey.

De-Stress dinner guidelines
The smallest meal of the day
Try and eat a little less in the evenings and go to bed a little hungry so that you have an appetite for breakfast the next morning. It takes around 10 minutes for your stomach to signal fullness to the brain, so give that a chance to happen. Try and eat between 6.30 and 8 p.m. if you can.

Eat protein and vegetables
Having adequate protein (see page 98) in the evenings is essential. Protein contains amino acids that your body needs for the rebuilding processes it performs at night and it can only get some of these directly from food.

Limit starchy carbs
If you choose to include grains, beans and potatoes in your diet, have them at breakfast or lunch to avoid the insulin surge that can lead to weight gain around the middle. If you're eating out, avoid pasta, potatoes and the bread basket and have an extra side order of vegetables instead.

Avoid puddings and sweets
Save these for a very occasional treat. Eating sugar, crisps and chocolate in the evening promotes an insulin surge and stimulates a blood-sugar spike before bed. See the best fruit in the lists above as sweet alternatives, to help soothe the brain through serotonin and GABA production.

Smart dining out
If you're going out to dinner, opt for a light salad starter and avoid dessert, choosing protein and plenty of veg where you can. The best starters 'whet the appetite' and stimulate digestive juices so you can better assimilate the nutrients in your main course. These are usually bitter or sour foods that stimulate the pancreas to produce bile, which helps you digest the meal to come.

Great choices of bile-promoting foods include grapefruit, olives, watercress, artichoke, chicory, parsley and radicchio. Avoid creamy dressings and instead liven up your meat, fish, pulses and vegetables with olive oil, fresh lemon juice, herbs such as parsley, unsalted butter, garlic, spices, mustard, vinegar and freshly made dressings.

If you overdo it

Remember, we evolved to eat a little less on some days, a bit more on others and occasionally, a lot. If you ate a little more than usual last night, know your body will cope and that it's good to let it know it isn't in the stress of a famine sometimes!

Visit my site www.charlottewattshealth.com and see the Guide to Healthy Take-away and Dining Out Options.

How you have dinner

Here's the ideal De-Stress dinner routine, with options depending on the amount of time you have to devote to it.

- Even if you feel stressed and hungry when you get in, take just one minute to first sit and arrive in your breath and your home. Then you're in a place to be mindful of what you're doing (even if it's chopping vegetables), how you're feeling, and to invite your breath to slow down. If you feel you need to eat something as you prepare dinner, have some almonds or half an avocado with some lemon juice and black pepper; these provide fats that will satisfy you without ruining your appetite.

- Play some classical music when you get home – if you have some Bach or Brahms, great, but anything soothing helps you relax into your evening.

- Set the table for dinner in an appealing way, with a simple bunch of flowers or a low candle to make the meal an event.

- Truly relax, eat slowly and chew while you eat: this helps tell your body you're full and aids complete digestion.

- Wait 10–15 minutes before going for something sweet or for second helpings. If you really want seconds, ask yourself, 'How will this make me feel in half an hour?' Will you feel bloated and stuffed? Do you want to go to sleep feeling like that? If the answer is that you're simply still hungry, have more vegetables and a little protein.

Those stressy habits resolved

- If you're having wine with dinner, choose sulphate-free – preferably organic – and stick to a small glass.

- If you're a TV eater, dinner away from the box might take time to get used to. Try and start with one or two nights a week and gradually build up to every night.

- Once you've finished eating, chat or listen to others (or the radio) or read a book, for at least ten minutes before opting for a second helping or for pudding. This will give your body enough time to register satiety and fullness.

- If you fancy something sweet, try some seasonal fruit with Greek yoghurt or a square or two of dark chocolate (unless chocolate keeps you awake).

Troubleshooting

Explore these ideas for solving common sleep problems, alongside other De-Stress measures:

Problem: You can't calm down before bed.

Solution: Use 'sleep teas' such as chamomile, valerian and hops, lemon balm, passion flower. Make sure you get enough sunlight during the day for vitamin D, needed for correct calcium and magnesium utilization, and ensure you eat plenty of the sulphur foods on page 100 to ensure full vitamin D production. If your brain just won't switch off, get into the habit of writing down persistent thoughts in a notebook or diary.

Try a yoga nidra CD/audio download (see www.charlottewattshealth. com): this is the 'yoga of sleep' and is a guided, full-body relaxation that works for many people who find it difficult to relax, or who wake in the night. Celery is a traditional sleep remedy and a soothing celery soup can help (see chapter 5, Stressed and Wired, for more on celery).

Problem: You wake suddenly in the small hours.

Solution: Daytime blood-sugar highs and lows mean difficulty sustaining levels throughout the night, which causes a hypoglycaemic crash around 4 a.m. The survival reaction, an adrenaline surge, stops you slipping into a coma but can leave you suddenly awake and fearful and with a racing mind. Addressing daytime stress and blood-sugar issues gets to the root cause.

This can also apply to those who have disrupted sleep patterns caused by air travel or shift work, whose stress levels are known to be much higher. Have a bedtime snack – slow-release carbohydrate foods such as apples, oatcakes or celery help to keep up blood-glucose levels throughout sleep. Turn the alarm clock to face the other way – seeing the time is stimulating and could lead to more anxiety about the amount of sleep you're missing (probably less than you think!). Come to any mindfulness practice to accept where you are, and appreciate the feeling of being cocooned in bed, rather than focusing on the negative.

Our Stress Suits give us clues about what we need in the evening, especially when that can differ wildly from what we *want*.

Daily gratitude practice

To help us appreciate life and release our minds from grasping for something 'better' than what we believe we already have, a gratitude practice can bring us to a place of compassion with each breath and has been shown to reduce stress levels.[12] Each night before you go to sleep, simply think of or write down three things for which you feel grateful, and process the day's thoughts with a positive spin.

Try to do this even if you just don't feel that thankful – the signals still get through to your brain. Gratitude can often come less easily than grumbling, but continual practice has us noticing the little things in life that make us happy – and it releases all that energy used up hankering after 'grass is greener' fantasies. Sometimes just breathing and getting through a tough day is enough!

Help for your specific Stress Suit		
	You may find that you...	Best single change you could make
Stressed and Wired	can't stop 'doing' and then just can't get to sleep	Make time to do a full, 15-minute calming activity to retrain your nervous system and mind.
Stressed and Tired	feel shattered when you get home but then come awake around 9 p.m.	Aim for eight hours' sleep nightly and de-stressing in the day to prioritize quality sleep. Do a gentle early evening yoga practice.
Stressed and Cold	feel sluggish in the evening but still feel unrefreshed after sleep	Don't overheat your house or bedroom, so you stay alert (but calm) until the time you fully prepare for bed.
Stressed and Bloated	bloat after dinner, or feel gassy in the evening	Ensure dinner is light enough to digest and mindfully eaten to aid full absorption. Lying-down yoga twists can help.
Stressed and Sore	notice that inflammatory conditions worsen with poor sleep	Stay away from the inflammatory and excitatory sugars. Good-quality sleep gives your immune system the chance to clean up the day's invaders and repair areas of inflammation.
Stressed and Demotivated	sleep and sleep and sleep at the weekends	This might pay back a little of your sleep deficit, but ultimately it resets sleep cycles, making it harder to get up on Monday. Try to change perception so you can recognize the benefits of getting more sleep through the week.
Stressed and Hormonal	notice that any of the above get worse before a period, or menopausally	Prioritize De-Stress daily activities and make the evening time a sanctuary, particularly if you're used to clearing up and looking after others. Stay aware of how your breathing patterns signal that you're stressed.

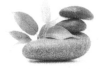

CHAPTER 14

Stress-Free Drinks and Snacks

*'Habit converts luxurious enjoyments
into dull and daily necessities.'*
ALDOUS HUXLEY

People often underestimate the amount of extra food, excess sugar, unhealthy fats and chemicals that sneaks into their diets as drinks and snacks. Our ancestors would have had the odd piece of fruit, some nuts and only water to drink. While the occasional 'treat' is fine, craving cycles and a need to turn constantly to snacks or sugary drinks is a sign that your main meals and lifestyle aren't supporting your energy needs. This chapter will help you move away from consuming the mindless snacks and drinks that are often simply a distraction.

LESS IS MORE

De-Stress Eating favours more sustaining meals over the 'little and often' ethos that has become popular recently and never gives the body a chance to experience true hunger, as well as putting a strain on digestion. Less snacking means feeling liberated from a sense that food is controlling you, especially when a mindfulness practice allows you to feel hunger as a natural sensation and not a hole to be immediately filled.

An American study looking at food habits during the last 30 years found that the number of times people ate in a day rose from 3.8 to 4.9.

During that time obesity rates doubled for adults and tripled for children.[1] The hormone ghrelin, which sets off hunger and a rumbling tummy, has been shown to be lower after meals containing fats and/or protein, while meals based on carbohydrates don't satisfy hunger in the same way and cause ghrelin to rise again quickly afterwards.[2] As high-carb, low-fat diets have been the mainstay of weight-loss recommendations for decades, this explains the continual need for snacking that has also become part of that picture.

Snacking between meals shouldn't be necessary if healthy fats and proteins are included in main meals; we should be able to go three or four hours without putting something into our mouths! In an ideal world we would have the freedom to eat when we're actually hungry, but work patterns often place restrictions on the timings of meals.

That time between lunch and dinner can be too long and for most of us, 4 p.m. usually signals a natural energy lull. This is the time when our metabolism is shifting from daytime activity gear to evening recovery mode, even though we're still expected to keep up energy and output.

If you have tired adrenal glands, the blood-sugar low common at this time can have you reaching for the brownies when you know dinner is still hours away. However, the right snack can pre-empt this and tide you through the journey home from work, keeping energy stable so you make good choices at dinner. The same can be said of mid-morning if your breakfast and lunch times feel too far apart.

DE-STRESS HEALTHY SNACKING

De-Stress Eating guidelines will help you crave less. By supporting your biochemistry, changing habits won't rely on willpower alone. It can be challenging as you move away from craving cycles (see chapter 7), but the following healthy snack guidelines can help you through the transition:

- Identify the healthiest snacks that you like and have them on hand when you might need them.

- Don't be fooled by marketing ploys: 23 almonds (a designated portion!) contains a quarter-teaspoon of sugar compared to one low-fat 'health' bar based on a 'slimming' cereal, which has around two teaspoons and a whole host of additives.

- Don't keep problem snacks in the house. This includes diet sodas or whatever you're drawn to for that hit, unless you're one of those unusual types who can have a tub of ice cream in the freezer and forget that it's there.

- If you feel intense hunger between meals or need to leave longer than four to five hours before your next meal, have a savoury snack that contains protein, such as almonds, to sate the driving hunger signals but not fuel a sweet tooth.

The following are the best snacks for energy, before exercise to ensure good fuel supplies, or even as emergency or lighter breakfasts:

De-Stress trail mix

Equal portions of any of the following:

- raw, unsalted nuts – choose and vary almonds, Brazils, hazelnuts, walnuts, pecans
- pumpkin and sunflower seeds
- dried unsweetened coconut
- unsulphured dried apricots, prunes, apple or mango – chopped to satisfy sweet cravings
- goji berries (reputed to support the adrenal glands)
- raw cocoa nibs can satisfy a chocolate craving and provide antioxidant polyphenols

Mix and store in an airtight container. A handful is a daily portion.

Vegetable sticks

Slice any raw vegetables that you like for crunch – celery, carrots, red peppers, cucumber and fennel all provide different nutrients. These can be stored in water with a little lemon juice for freshness and dipped in houmous, nut butters, mashed avocado or mackerel paté.

A hearty smoothie

Blend the following:

1. Half a large avocado
2. Half a tin of coconut milk (or make up 200ml (7 fl oz) from a block of coconut cream) or coconut water for an isotonic effect (see page 171)
3. 200ml (7 fl oz) freshly squeezed apple juice
4. A handful of berries – strawberries, blueberries, raspberries or a mixture (can be defrosted from frozen or blended while still partially frozen)
5. Optional ground almonds, whey, pea or hemp protein for a sports blend or breakfast choice

NOT SO 'GOOD FOR YOU'

Some food and drinks are smartly marketed as the healthy option, but aren't always so. When you've been De-Stress Eating for a few weeks you may begin to tune in to how sweet these foods taste and how they make you feel – probably not as satisfied as you expected. Be wary of the following foods that may be masquerading as healthy:

•   Drinks like hot chocolate, but also mocha coffees, iced coffee drinks and flavoured coffees with added syrups and hidden sugars.

•   Vitamin or fruit 'waters' and sports drinks – these are usually very high in sugar even though the label often states they are 'all natural'.

•   Diet soda – these have been shown to significantly increase waistlines in humans and confuse appetite signals.[3]

•   Fruit juices, especially from concentrate; imagine how much fruit – without fibre – is needed to make just one glass. Commercial orange juice can have more sugar than the equivalent volume of cola. Have the odd glass of freshly squeezed juice and dilute it by up to 50 per cent with water to reduce the sugar and cost. A high intake of fruit juice has been shown to be related to obesity and the benefits of vitamin C and antioxidants are outweighed by the sugar content. Choose the whole fruit instead.

- Commercial smoothies – even those with 'no added sugar' still pack a punch of fructose or other sugars from fruit. These can be preferable to juice, though, as they include more fibre, but check the label for added sugars; limit and choose dark fruits and berries for best blood-sugar balance.

- Processed, commercial cereals – even if it says 'added fibre' on the packet, this is often harsh, insoluble bran fibre, which can irritate the gut. So-called slimming cereals often have a high Glycaemic Index (GI) (releasing their sugars too quickly), and low-fat claims mean they can be like eating rather unsatisfying air.

- 'Slimming' snack bars are generally low on the fat and protein that might satisfy your appetite, while high in sugar. Their lightness and sweetness say it all: this won't satisfy you.

- Dried fruit can be a useful dietary component if used sparingly and seen as the concentrated sugar source that it is. Imagine the sugar in one grape – this amount is present in one raisin in a concentrated package. Dates are the worst choice, as their sugars hit the bloodstream as fast as pure glucose.

Beware sugar water

All sugary drinks have been shown to dull the palate and create a preference for sweet foods in just two weeks; it's always better to choose pure water, herbal or green tea.[4]

Best sweet alternatives

De-Stress Eating reduces habitual sweet tastes in your diet, but the following occasional healthy treats can be an alternative to giving in entirely on those more challenging or stressful days. Buy the best-quality products when you plan to eat something sweet and enjoy them without guilt:

- Dried mango, apricots, figs, prunes, apples – buy unsweetened and 'unsulphured' without the preservative sulphur dioxide, which can cause digestive discomfort.

- Stewed apples and plums sweetened with just a little honey.

- Baked apples – easy to fill with honey and cinnamon; can be kept for later as delicious sliced treats.

- Healthy snack bars – many of these are incredibly sweet as they are glued together with high-sugar dates or other syrupy stickiness. Look for those with nuts and the least amount of the sugars listed on page 107; beware the bar with a sugar source high up on the list.

- Oat-based biscuits or flapjacks can be the best occasional choice if you're going to succumb to the sugar/grain combo, as they release their sugars slowly.

Also see suggestions in chapter 7 (Understanding Cravings).

Chocolate

With a poll of 1,965 people showing that some women rate chocolate above sex and some men rate it above a spin in a sports car,[5] the suggestion to reduce it is made with caution! Chocolate is rich in the anti-inflammatory and heart-protective polyphenol antioxidants also found in wine and green tea,[6] but don't be fooled by talk of 'natural sugars' – chocolate is bitter and if it's sweet it contains sugar or a sweetener. Choose small amounts of high-quality chocolate to take advantage of the 'happy chemical' beta-endorphins that it helps the brain produce, although much of this effect is from the sugar and fat combination.[7]

De-Stress chocolate guidelines

- One small bar (40g/1½oz or so) of dark chocolate every few days is fine; try it flavoured with mint or orange oil, nuts, chilli or other spices. One study showed that 40g (1½oz) a day of dark chocolate helped people cope with stress.[8]

- A 40g (1½oz) bar of milk chocolate will contain not only dairy, but also as much as seven teaspoons of sugar compared to a three-teaspoon average for the same weight of 70 per cent cocoa dark chocolate.

- Five or six dark chocolate-covered Brazil nuts have more of the nut protein present, so they come with more flavour and satisfaction.

- Pay more and buy less. Quality over quantity can make you more of a healthy connoisseur than an unhealthy sugar addict.

- Raw chocolate has become popular because, unlike during commercial preparation, the beans aren't roasted, which means they retain much higher levels of antioxidants and have a less agitating caffeine effect; they are often made with coconut cream instead of dairy.

Fruit

Our ancestors ate fruit, which of course seems natural and healthy. Recommendations to eat two to three portions of fruit maximum a day can help keep your diet mainly savoury and keep sweet cravings under control. Apples and berries are particularly good fruit choices as they blunt the rise of digested sugars after a meal. This makes them a useful option if you're weaning off a dessert habit, but pick berries if you tend towards bloating, as apples (and potentially other fruit we use to make alcoholic drinks) easily ferment if eaten straight after protein.

Apples, apricots, cherries, oranges, plums (and also carrots) contain the soluble fibre pectin, which satisfies appetite by holding food in the stomach for longer. Pectin has also been shown to limit the amount of fat your cells can absorb to help curb damage from meals high in saturated fat. Grapes, mangoes, dried apricots, dried figs, dates, raisins, watermelon and bananas are high in sugar, particularly fructose, so they are the least healthy choices, but are still a good occasional choice if you're struggling with sweet cravings.

Nuts and seeds

Nuts may be high in anti-nutrients (nature is full of them to protect growing plants!) but they formed part of our hunter-gatherer ancestors' diets, so it's believed that we're more adapted to the lectins they contain. They provide crucial protein for vegetarians (and especially vegans), soluble fibre, minerals and essential oils.

Nuts contain immune-modulating properties (especially when eaten with their skin) and those who include them in their diet tend to have better weight management,[9] partly through appetite satisfaction.[10] Nuts also have a neutral acid-alkaline balance, making them a better source of starchy carbohydrates than grains.

THE IMPORTANCE OF HYDRATION

Like snacks, drinks have become a massive industry and yet it's easy to become dehydrated if we take in too little water through the most natural route: whole vegetables and fruit. Insufficient hydration impacts all aspects of health, but it's felt most obviously as fatigue. Bloating is also common, as your system holds on to the little it's receiving. Hydration is crucial during exercise for endurance and coordination; dehydration triggers histamine production and inflammation, with muscle performing badly and becoming more prone to injury.

However, the 'two litres a day' message is now being refuted in many scientific circles, replaced by a recommendation for drinking when thirsty and hydrating from fluid and mineral-rich vegetables and fruit.[11] This helps avoid the mineral loss and strain on our kidneys that too much water alone can bring. Too high a water intake can produce hyponatremia, or low sodium levels in the blood, with symptoms of confusion, fatigue, irritability and muscle cramps.

When you're generally hydrated, with good mineral balances, it's easier to connect to your natural thirst mechanism. This kicks in when we lose about 1–2 per cent of our body's water (mild dehydration) and will vary according to how much exercise we're doing and how hot and/or dry our environment is; air conditioning and air travel definitely qualify as dehydrating.

Stress and disordered breathing patterns can also cause more moisture loss and if more than 2 per cent of normal water volume is lost, true dehydration occurs, with possible dry skin and loss of appetite. Timing is crucial: many people drink too little water between meals, providing insufficient liquid with which to produce digestive juices and keep the bowel hydrated. Not chewing enough prompts drinking with meals to lubricate food for swallowing, but this can dilute stomach acid, reducing digestive efficacy further. Drink water between meals and sip only a little with food.

Better hydration in your diet

Simply increasing the amount of water in a dehydrated body can be like watering a dry pot plant: you see the water go straight through without being absorbed. Try these methods to help rehydrate effectively:

* Increase your intake of vegetables and fruit, as these contain potassium and sugars that help the water they contain enter cells more easily than water alone, while soluble fibre hydrates the bowel. The stews on page 123 are particularly effective for upping your intake and supporting the gut lining.

* If your diet has been low in fruit and veg, high in caffeine and added stress, dehydration-related symptoms such as constipation, headaches and dry skin may have been the result. Increase your liquid intake slowly, substituting sugary snacks for two glasses of half-apple juice (freshly squeezed 'cloudy' version), half-water for the first few weeks of the De Stress Eating plan, then tapering off to replace with water and the recommended fluids.

* As an isotonic fluid, coconut water contains the same balance of minerals as our own blood plasma and can be helpful for replenishing stores lost during exercise.[12] It is a better health choice than sugary commercial isotonic sports drinks, supporting good performance and recovery.

- Drink filtered water with lemon juice for alkalizing with the fewest impurities; filter water at home and carry in a stainless steel or BPA-free plastic bottle for the day.

- Herbal teas are an excellent way to hydrate, especially if you make your own from fresh mint, fennel seeds or fresh ginger and lemon – they are also caffeine-free. Add cinnamon to sweeten and a tiny bit of honey, only as you're weaning yourself off sugar.

- Spice teas taste great and also supply the properties of the spices, especially when made without a teabag. A chai Indian tea mix typically includes any of the following in varying amounts: cardamom, cinnamon, ginger, fennel seeds, peppercorn, liquorice and cloves. Make a simple blend to your taste and add a quarter of a teaspoon of it per small mug of water and drink the spices.

- Rooibush or redbush tea is non-caffeinated African tea that is the best substitute for a regular caffeinated 'cuppa'. It comes in flavoured versions too, like vanilla, chai and Earl Grey.

CAFFEINE

Anthropologists believe that we've been consuming caffeine in low levels in green tea since the Stone Age.[13] It's an extremely reliable drug, delivering a quick jolt to the central nervous system for the increased wakefulness, mental acuity, alertness and focus many of us love. But this is going for a quick fix: it doesn't remove the need for rest, it just masks the sensations of tiredness. As a stimulant, caffeine stimulates the HPAA (see page 9) to energize and raise blood sugar.[14]

The reliance on this unnatural energy comes as caffeine binds to adenosine receptors in the brain, keeping these energy-stimulators revved up and stopping the ability of the blood vessels to dilate and let our bodies feel oxygenated and sleepy. This isn't good before bed, and if you consider that our bodies are preparing these retiring processes from 4 p.m. onwards, caffeine isn't advised beyond around 2–3 p.m.

Studies have consistently failed to show that caffeine causes dehydration in moderate amounts,[15] but it's best avoided if it's making you feel more stressed. For some of us, though, high-quality coffee or tea can provide a healthy lift if kept to two cups maximum a day – for example one after breakfast and/or lunch.[16]

If you're having a shop-bought coffee ask for a single shot, so as not to over-stimulate your system. If you're used to having a cup of coffee or tea before breakfast, save this until you have food in your stomach. That can temper the adrenaline response to caffeine and make later crashes less likely.

Lowering caffeine slowly

As with most drugs, physical dependency on caffeine comes from the dopamine 'reward high' it produces.[17] Withdrawal can lead to symptoms like headaches, fatigue, moodiness and constipation. These generally occur after 12 hours without caffeine, peak after 24–48 hours and last for up to a week.

Knowing this helps us to see the reactions for what they are and plan how to manage withdrawal alongside sugar reduction and endorphin support (see page 95). Aim to get high caffeine intake down to two cups a day, but if you also have a high-sugar diet, prioritize lowering this first. Then taper off caffeine to a level where you don't see sugar cravings worsen before your natural energy levels increase. Fewer stimulants can eventually mean fewer sugar cravings, but this can take weeks to settle.

Natural cortisol balance

Liquorice tea is the best alternative to caffeine for those who have become Stressed and Tired and struggle to maintain natural energy without stimulants. It keeps cortisol circulating when it's low,[18] so it's good for a natural energy boost in the morning – but not past early afternoon. This effect is so good, though, that liquorice tea is contra-indicated for those with high blood pressure.[19] Commercial blends in tea bags are readily available or liquorice root flakes can be added to water or herbal tea.

Caffeine withdrawal can come with extreme energy slumps as your brain chemistry resensitizes to using its own natural energy. Plan for this and reduce on a Friday to give yourself a seriously laid-back weekend. Bring down any sugar or sweeteners in tea or coffee gradually beforehand, replacing with cinnamon if this suits you.

The stimulants theobromine and theophylline are still present in decaffeinated drinks, so they will create some stimulation. Choose good-quality water-filtered decaf if going this route, but it's better to stick to green tea or herbal teas. Tea and coffee can be sprayed with huge amounts of chemicals, so choose organic.

How much caffeine are you getting?

About 200–300mg of caffeine a day is generally recommended as the safe upper limit to avoid the insomnia, anxiety, nausea and accelerated heart rate that comes with overstimulation. When you consider that a 'grande'-sized coffee from a well-known coffee chain has as much as 350mg of caffeine per cup, you can suddenly see why there are so many highly agitated folk about. For some, though, symptoms can be set off even by a weak cup of tea, so monitor your own reactions.

300mg caffeine roughly equates to:

- Four average cups or three average-sized mugs of instant coffee

- Three average cups of brewed coffee

- Six average cups of tea

- Eight cans of regular cola

- Four cans of an 'energy drink'

- Eight standard 50g/1½oz bars (or 400g/14oz) of plain chocolate

Stimulating and soothing green tea

Green tea is a great replacement for stronger black tea and coffee – like all tea, it has high levels of protective antioxidant catechins [20], which counter the overstimulating effects of the small amount of caffeine present.[21] Experiment with different brands and varieties, only brew for 30 seconds to avoid a bitter taste and try chai and other flavoured versions if you aren't keen at first. The Japanese Genmaicha and Sencha varieties are delicious. Green tea also contains a substance called L-Theanine, known to have calming and focusing effects on body and mind.[22]

ALCOHOL

Drinking less than two units a day of red wine has been shown to be a contributory component in lowering heart disease and obesity risk through its potent antioxidant resveratrol.[23] Wine was a prominent feature of the healthiest Mediterranean diet of Crete, where it was estimated to add a year to life expectancy when combined with other components such as plenty of vegetables, fruit, olive oil and garlic.[24]

Straying above the UK's recommended 14 weekly units for women and 21 for men can soon negate these benefits, though, especially if you're clocking them all up on a Friday night, putting dangerous pressure on your liver. Remember, one unit is one 175ml (6 fl oz) glass of wine, not a large, half-bottle-sized glassful. It's not only binge-drinking but also that continual drip-feeding of daily alcohol to amounts above healthy limits that has been shown to increase risks of breast cancer, heart disease, diabetes and osteoporosis,[25] as well as damaging memory and slowing reaction times.[26]

As a sugar source, alcohol has the same effects as any other, raising insulin and turning on fat storage by increasing fatty deposits in the liver. The intoxication it causes is, by its very definition, toxic to the body and causes damage to all the liver's detoxification pathways. The liver works overtime to eject it, but the alcohol itself depletes the very substances needed to speed it out of the body, especially those required for energy and dealing with stress and blood-sugar balance, such as B vitamins, vitamin C, magnesium, zinc and chromium.

For many, alcohol may seem essential for 'switching off'. This is because its first response is to relax us by heightening the relaxing brain chemical GABA (see page 53).[27,28] This becomes a cycle where the brain starts to need alcohol to pick up the GABA, and without it we can then become tense, anxious and unable to sleep. Using alcohol to help sleep is a false economy: the GABA rush does stupefy and relax us at first, but then lowered levels throughout the night can impair sleep and jolt us awake in the small hours.

Reducing alcohol intake can create a phase where less GABA (and dopamine) is available to the brain, and you may feel this agitation and inability to self-soothe and maintain a good mood while your brain resensitizes to accessing its own stores. This can be difficult, especially for Stressed and Demotivated types, but it's crucial at this stage not to turn to other sugar sources to replace this effect and 'normalize'. That simply replaces one addictive cycle with another. Women may also experience more alcohol cravings premenstrually, as will anyone during times of stress for soothing self-medication.

De-Stress alcohol guidelines

- If having a glass of wine with a meal several times a week is your treat, stick to that and avoid other sugar sources.

- Quality is key: spend more and buy less to become a connoisseur rather than a guzzler. You can even encourage your friends to do the same. With red wine, the deeper the colour, the higher the antioxidant count, with the best amounts seen in Merlot, Cabernet Sauvignon and Chianti. Rioja and Pinot Noir are in the middle and the least benefit comes from Côtes du Rhône.

- Champagne or dry white wines contain less sugar than sweeter red or white wines: they are the best choice for those wanting the occasional celebratory drink while staying off sweet tastes.

- Gin or vodka with soda and a twist of lime are the best low-sugar choices, providing water for hydration and avoiding the problem sugars or sweeteners in mixers. Whisky, vodka, gin and rum have little sugar when drunk on their own, so switch to an occasional shot on the rocks.

- Beers, dessert wines, fortified wines (e.g. sherry, port), sweet wines and brandy all have high sugar content, so avoid these.

- Grain-based alcohols like beer, ales and vodka may affect those with grain intolerance.

- For everyone, good liver support is essential when reducing any addictive cycles. See pages 100 and 110, and ensure good hydration.

See www.charlottewattshealth.com for a chart to help identify and reduce alcohol intake.

Social lubrication

Britain is a nation of drinkers and many people can feel extreme social pressure from friends and work colleagues not to appear 'boring' or different. Some people can feel threatened when others reduce how much they drink or give up alcohol altogether, but a growing number of us are doing so, especially as we hit our late thirties and beyond and the hangovers get worse. Learning to go out without drinking to excess is a mindful skill to be learned – a reconditioning that takes practice but ultimately leads to enjoying yourself without a 'pay-back'.

Consider whether you have a tendency to drink alone to numb yourself or combat 'bad stress' and explore. Never drink on an empty stomach and always ensure you have good protein before a drink to curb blood-sugar spikes and help detoxify the alcohol. Eggs are especially good as they contain high levels of cysteine, a sulphur amino acid that helps break down alcohol – this is the reason they are an age-old hangover cure in many cultures.

Avoiding friends who drink or situations that revolve around alcohol can help while you change the biochemical effects, but it's ultimately avoiding the problem. If you're out to dinner or in the pub chatting, pay attention to how much you're drinking. It's easy to keep knocking back a newly filled glass, especially in a culture in which drinking more is lauded.

Alternate alcoholic drinks with sparkling water with lemon (not sugary soft drinks or juice), to both support your liver and reduce alcohol intake. Learn to say no and not feel pressured. It's your choice to drink or not, and it's not appropriate for others to badger, cajole or bully you into having more than you want – that's a form of social stress and if it's in your life it needs to be nipped in the bud with an assertive 'no thanks' and no need to justify. You may need to discuss your choice with friends away from the pub.

If you drink to any level nearing alcoholism (consult your GP to define this), do not give up alcohol suddenly as that can be very dangerous. Safe withdrawal is known as *tapering* and should be done under the supervision of a medical professional.

Snacks and drinks by Stress Suit		
	You may find that you...	Best single change you could make
Stressed and Wired	rely on a barrage of sugar, caffeine and/ or alcohol to stay 'up'	Allow rest when your body and brain need recovery, including backing off the stimulants systematically.
Stressed and Tired	can't make it to the next meal without craving something sweet	Explore when you might need a well-chosen snack to level out long-term blood-sugar imbalances. Use liquorice tea to energize naturally.
Stressed and Cold	don't quite feel satisfied after meals and, although bloated, still want more	Drink a cup of strong peppermint tea about 20 minutes before a meal, to stimulate stomach acid and bile for best nutrient absorption.
Stressed and Bloated	end up snacking later as you avoid larger meals, especially when stressed	Avoid drinking an hour either side of meals. Mix dried mint, ginger, cumin and fennel seeds for a post-meal digestive tea.
Stressed and Sore	aren't sure what's going on; you just seem so reactive to different foods	Ensure good hydration levels; reduce sugar and caffeine. Add turmeric to spice tea mix and choose green tea as a mild caffeine source.
Stressed and Demotivated	end up eating sugar or comfort foods for no good reason	Find the right treats for you – for example, daily dark chocolate. That way you'll know you've had a treat, while you address other aspects.
Stressed and Hormonal	want more sugar before your period	'Detox' teas can be a quick and easy extra liver support. Prioritize reducing alcohol, as it can raise oestrogen and is known to be a breast cancer risk.

PART III

Living the
De-Stress Effect

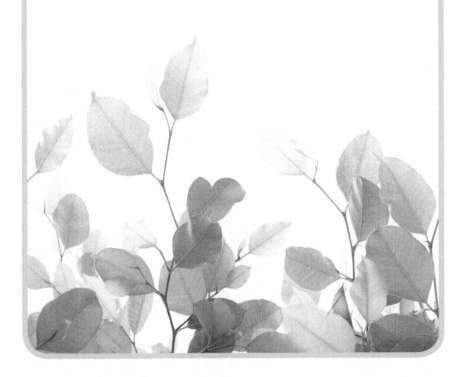

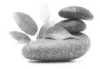

CHAPTER 15

The Mindfulness Practices

*'Do not use your mind to overcome by force: you
must fit into the ancient grooves naturally.'*
HERMIT OF LOTUS FLOWER PEAK

Practising mindfulness as formal meditation creates a seed to grow into our daily lives, helping us understand ourselves better and make choices from a more open and less reactive place. Research has shown that regular mindfulness practice of just 10 minutes minimum a day can affect our neural pathways (brain chemistry) and change our perspective; this includes the naturally conscious nature of an embodied yoga practice, which is explored in the next chapter.

As discussed in chapter 3, mindfulness is gathering interest and respect from Western philosophers and researchers, as our culture tends to feed comparison, self-criticism and judgement. For those who meditate it isn't news that cultivating a more kind, loving and gentle attitude towards ourselves ripples out into the world, feeding back to us as part of the community.

This connection to others fosters an easier social engagement, which integrates higher (more rational) and lower (more emotionally reactive) brain functions to feel reason and instinct fall into smooth patterns of communication. Practitioners feel increasing:

- Freedom from negative thoughts and emotions
- Greater awareness of the richness and beauty of everyday things
- Calmness and a sense of spaciousness
- Sensitivity and responsiveness to life so we make better choices
- Letting go of preoccupation with thoughts, feelings and bodily sensations

There are many practice routes to moving away from brain chatter to body awareness and space to feel calm. These work as a web of tools to offer the right flavour of focus at the right time for you. The essence of mindfulness is curiosity and exploration. Seeing what unfolds and meeting it with compassion is a continually changing and evolving journey. Each practice will feel different – of the moment!

MEETING VULNERABILITY

Being alone and quiet in the present moment asks us to be open and vulnerable, which can seem a scary place to be. Stress can have us locked in a hard, defensive place and letting that go to soften can sometimes feel uncomfortable. Courage is the fuel we need to allow an expansive feel to our inner worlds.

Focusing on our hearts is a helpful light in the fog. Placing a hand on your heart whenever you need to can remind you that you're real and here, and help you direct breathing to feel supported. If being still causes rising anxiety for you at the start, a moving practice like yoga can help provide the focus that your brain needs. Our brains have a built-in desire to seek stimulation and while breath focus can provide that for some, others need body engagement, particularly when training awareness.

Ultimately, all meditation is moving towards a state of complete absorption or zen, but most of us were conditioned from a young age to strive for targets, goals and efficiency, so we can panic a tad when these are removed. The primal seeking desire for mates, food and other things we need to survive now manifests as patterns like sugar addiction and compulsive eBay shopping when we're stressed.

Remove these negative coping methods and the brain can seek something, anything – even if that is negative and churning thoughts. This is one of the reasons why meditation raises cortisol levels for some when they begin practising. Another is that we have to work cognitively at the practice before it becomes familiar, so that it can be stimulating before it becomes quieting.

We all have individual neurological make-up and reaction patterns – through conditioning in our ancestors' lives (genetic) and learned within our own. But we are all here together and you can feel some comfort from knowing that anything you feel isn't unusual, strange or a sign you're doing something wrong.

As the esteemed yoga teacher Judith Lasater says, *'Life is difficult, we have a choice whether to struggle.'* Struggle is one response to challenge but we can also choose to step back. The more we can meet external and internal agitation with *equanimity* – the quality of non-reaction – the easier life can be.

The middle way

In her book *Rewire Your Brain for Love*, neuropsychologist Marsha Lucas explains how mindfulness helps both integrate and balance 'your logical, linear, language-y left hemisphere and your non-verbal, "whole-picture", raw, spontaneous-emotion, stress-modulating right hemisphere'. Too much right hemisphere and life seems like a barrage of raw, unmodulated experience, so we respond with withdrawal, but when the left can stay present we can be curious instead and approach.

Too much left and we can be dominated by mind-chatter and unable to experience the fullness of life around us. Lucas says that 'if your left brain and right brain are working as a balanced team, each bringing their own strengths… You can do your thinking and it'll be informed by what your body's reacting to and what your emotional brew is cooking up.'

With meditators showing larger grey-matter volumes than non-meditators in brain areas associated with emotional regulation and response control, as well as increased attention, self-esteem, visual perception, socio-emotional wellbeing, sensory processing, learning, memory, cardiovascular health and anti-ageing, it's a question of why wouldn't ya?

This *neuroplasticity*, or ability to change neural pathways and old grooves, is ultimately what has us handling our lives with more ease, grace, kindness and patience. It's what meditators have known for thousands of years and Western science is catching up on.

MEETING YOUR MONKEY MIND THROUGH MEDITATION

The Buddhist term 'monkey mind' describes the ever chattering and leaping tendencies of our brain, and is also so called because this internal chaos comes from the brain's most evolved neomammalian or primate part. We can feed our monkey mind by giving ourselves a hard time about it, often most ironically when meditating.

Yet we need to have a little gratitude for these tendencies because they kept our ancestors alive with the vigilance to stay safe and now they are always running along in the background, waiting for the chance to save the day. As Rick Hanson says in his illuminating book *Buddha's Brain*, 'Sensations, emotions, desires, and other mind-objects are *supposed* to attract attention so you'll respond to them. Letting them roll by without hopping on board just isn't natural.'

> 'Do you have the patience to wait until your
> mud settles and the water is clear? Can you remain
> unmoving until the right action arises by itself?'
> LAO TZU

When we meditate, rather than focusing on 'emptying the mind', which can be a forceful act in a busy brain, we can shift this perspective to 'inviting letting go', which can pacify rather than alert the monkeys:

- Cultivate non-reaction. The basis of meditation isn't pushing away thoughts but acknowledging them without getting involved or following stories that arise. This helps us to simply step to one side, become the observer and nurture non-attachment, not letting individual thoughts become larger stories in our minds.

- We'll always wander away from the present – it's our nature. Ruminating on the past or projecting into the future is where we go when we aren't in the present moment. It's an ingrained habit to follow thoughts, feelings (and thoughts about a feeling, feelings about a thought), dilemmas, worries, etc. Watch tendencies for self-doubt, anger, resentment, restlessness and boredom that steal you away from the here and now. These *hindrances* are natural: 'Let them all come and let them all go.'

- Self-compassion and patience create the anchor or *grounding* that we need to foster awareness. A useful phrase (again from Judith Lasater) to say to yourself is '*how human of me* to get distracted/tell myself off/get bored'. That helps us to let go and not create criticism from noticing our tendencies. Everyone has these challenges – you aren't alone and are no worse (or better) than anyone else.

- Practise gratitude by thanking the chattering monkey voices for looking out for you and invite them to calm through your breath (see pages 30–31). This is both simple and complicated. Don't judge your practice, it is what it is and it will always differ – some days an easy flow, some days like wading through treacle or feeling like you're in the trenches. Whether meditation feels easy or difficult, it will always benefit you.[1,2,3]

- When we meditate and in life generally, acceptance is the route to being with any nature of feeling that arises. This isn't putting up with things we shouldn't, but rather easing off energy wasted on fight and turmoil to accept that trying to control things keeps us from living with ease.

Kind discipline

Our mindfulness practice is to notice when we have 'left the building' and guide ourselves back with consistency and patience – kindly and steadily, like a shepherd tending to a flock, or leading back a child that's wandered away. The discipline is to practise wakefulness for when we might stray, then simply inhale to gather in and exhale back into awareness without self-criticism. We guide back over and over, as many times as we wander.

Treat yourself well – get comfortable

Although most meditation images show a sitting position, if you don't often or easily sit cross-legged, this can initially create more tension in the neck, shoulders, chest, back or hips and dominate the experience.

It's better to be fully supported in a way that allows the whole body to rest and the chest to open easily, or you can feel like you're swimming upstream rather than flowing with the river. There are enough undercurrents to meet without adding more! This preparation is part of our practice – we can be used to holding ourselves in uncomfortable positions and sometimes can't recognize where we need to let go physically.

1. Lying down with a folded towel under your head and pillows under your knees allows full diaphragmatic breathing as the chest is fully supported.

2. If you're happy sitting cross-legged, sit on a cushion or folded blanket to raise hips above knees and lift up through the spine with the chin tucked a little into your throat.

3. Sitting on a chair is an option for a longer practice, if tightness in the hips creates tension in the knees or chest-opening feels tense. Support the lower back with a cushion for ease, sitting upright if you need to and lifting the back of the skull rather than the chin.

4. For a shorter 'stay' – time spent practicing – just sitting where you are (desk, train) and lifting through the spine can create a more spacious passage for your breath.

Ultimately, through practice and help from yoga to strengthen postural support, sitting upright creates a sharpening of focus via internal feedback to nerves in the brain stem – the *reticular formation* – involved in consciousness and wakefulness. 'Sitting up straight' is a signal to alertness.

Breath by breath, moment to moment

Breath is an anchor in mindfulness because it's something we can always feel, mostly have a neutral (neither good nor bad) feeling towards and it's happening every second we are alive. It roots us in the present; we can't breathe in the past, nor is it possible to take a breath into the future.

Many body responses are beyond our control and happen without us noticing, but breathing is unusual in that it's both autonomic (automatic) and within our control. Consciously calming our breath sends signals to the nervous system that we're safe and can come down from the primed-for-danger alert state that has the heart racing and the jaw clenching. When we don't notice such stress signs (and those from breathing itself on page 39) we miss the opportunity to engage directly with our nervous system and self-soothe via breath influence – including before eating.

Daily practice of mindful breathing can prepare you to cope with the coming day or help you let go of its pressures at the end.[4] Every little helps: two minutes achieved is better than planning for 20 minutes and then doing nothing – creating the pointless stress of failure. See page 188 for more information on breathing and taking this into a mindful movement practice.

Practice: Mindfulness of breathing

Feeling our breath within our physical body can help still the commentary or narration of our lives that can be running along in the background.

1. Firstly, sit or lie completely comfortably, close your eyes and let your whole body settle. Fidget if you need to for a few moments, so you feel you're in a place where you can sustain stillness and be with any feelings that arise.

2. Simply observe your breath like a tide: naturally flowing in and out with no expectation or imposition, right to the end. Be aware of every subtlety with all of your senses in every single moment, trusting your breath, not looking for anything particular to happen and accepting any feelings as they arise.

3. Notice all of the sensations: your breath across your top lip and nostrils, cool as it comes in, warm as it leaves; the rise and fall of belly and chest; knowing that every breath affects every single cell in your body.

Another variation of the Buddhist meditation mindfulness of breathing (Anapanasati) uses counting down from 10 to one to provide a stable focal point and occupy that chatty left brain. It can be used as a guide into stillness any time, or as an interception to focus when stress arises:

1. Begin counting 10 on the inhalation, 10 to one on the exhalation. Continue counting the full breath cycle like this down to one, and then start again.

2. If your mind wanders or you lose count, simply start again at 10. If you begin counting automatically without full focus on the breath, start again.

3. Continue until you feel sufficiently attuned to your breath to follow without counting – you can always come back.

Metta Bhavana

Metta Bhavana is one of the core Buddhist meditations. It translates (from Pali) as *Metta* meaning loving-kindness and *Bhavana* meaning to cultivate or develop. With the Western tendencies for self-criticism and judging inner voices, this practice is gathering interest and respect from ideologies and researchers.

Metta is an allowing, rather than a pushing, of feelings of friendship, benevolence, friendliness, goodwill, compassion, love, gentleness and kindness. It's simply bringing these qualities together to create a warm-hearted and non-violent landscape in which to hold the feelings that arise, even when they are challenging.

At any stage you can offer 'may I/they be well and happy'. As Hanson says in *Buddha's Brain*: 'If compassion is the wish that beings not suffer, then kindness is the wish that they be happy' – and that includes you.

Practice: Metta Bhavana meditation

Find a comfortable position (sitting or lying) and focus your attention inwards to your breath until you feel you've 'dropped-in' and arrived at a receptive place. Then move through each of the following 'stages of attention' outlined below. It can help to set a pleasant-sounding timer (e.g. through a meditation timer app such as the Insight Timer) to signal when to move to the next stage so you don't feel the urge to look at a clock and can simply 'be' with the expanse of time.

You can start with whatever length of time works for you to build up feeling safe with the practice; even two to three minutes per stage will help you feel the effects, with five to 10 minutes on each making a deeper connection.

Practice whenever you can: in the morning helps set the tone for good interactions with others, before bed promotes happy and nourishing dreams.

1. Yourself – visualize bringing peace and calm to your whole body. You can imagine kindness flowing in as a radiant light and feel it breathing in and out from your heart and opening up into all parts of your body.

2. A good friend – move your focus to someone with whom you have an easy connection and with whom you feel you have mutual, unconditional support. Hold the feelings of their good qualities, your connection and how they make you feel.

3. A neutral person – take your attention to someone you neither particularly like or dislike; it could be someone you had a fleeting communication with or see around. Reflect on their humanity, how they too are deserving of love and kindness, and wish them well.

4. A person with whom you have difficulty – move to someone you've formed a negative opinion of – someone who causes a reaction in you, but not one so difficult that you become immersed in past trauma or thoughts of a complicated situation. Try not to get caught up in the reactions of your judgement, but feel how you can find a way to wish that person happiness and accept that they too are worthy of kindness.

5. All four persons above together – bring all four subjects together to feel the differing types of connection meld as a community. Open your heart to feel the non-discrimination of compassion.

6. All beings everywhere – feel your heart opening to expand out with waves of love; feel that there is space for everyone to receive kindness and feel yourself as part of that larger community and expanse – a giving and receiving.

7. Spend some moments gathering yourself back in to draw your practice to a close. Focus back onto yourself if you need to, even bringing a hand onto your heart to gain a sense of your physical self.

A trial showed that the ability to feel mindfulness, self-compassion and resilience following a Metta-based retreat improved significantly in a group of 44 human services professionals,[5] so the ripple effect of this more loving attitude could really plant the seeds of greater working environments for others.

Walking kindness

Heather Mason, founder of the Minded Institute says, '*Mindfulness meditation can be challenging to those who struggle with rumination and constant anxious thinking. There are, however, ways to help a person develop enough calm in order to be able to better grapple with mindfulness.*

'*One of my favourites is to combine loving-kindness meditation with walking meditation, where specific phrases are recited mentally. This really helps to relax the mind and to ease in positive feeling to those who would normally struggle with loving thoughts. Simply walk with no need to get anywhere, paying attention to the sensations of body movement up from the ground.'* Heather suggests repeating, 'May I be happy and peaceful' as we lift the foot and 'May I be healthy and at ease' when we place the foot.

Mindful interceptions

If our minds are churning and directing stress back at us, it's helpful to draw on mindful exercises that help create space and a less negative perspective.[6,7]

Practice: The three-step breathing space

This practice is outlined in *The Mindful Way through Depression* by Mark Williams, John Teasdale, Zindel Segal and Jon Kabat-Zinn. It's a technique used in MBSR (Mindfulness-based Stress Reduction) and MBCT (Mindfulness-based Cognitive Therapy) courses, which offer tools for dealing with stress and its effects on daily life.

The breathing space can be practised whenever you need a less stress-inducing alternative to an ingrained, autopilot response. It can be practised over as short a period as three breaths (in any position), as a lifeline to a calmer state, or at the beginning of a meditation when connecting feels difficult. There are three distinct steps to follow:

1. Awareness: close your eyes if feels right, or settle your gaze onto one spot if not. Investigate and explore how things are right now, even asking yourself: *What is my experience right now? What thoughts are here? What emotions? What bodily sensations?* Acknowledge all aspects of the experience – wanted and unwanted – without judgement.

2. Gathering: gently draw your awareness into your breath, observing each part of the inhalation and exhalation. Experience the physical sensations of breathing in your abdomen.

3. Expanding: now expand your field of awareness out from your belly, so it includes a sense of your body as a whole, including your posture and facial expressions. You may want to say on the out-breath: 'It's okay… whatever it is, it's already here: let me feel it'. Move this expanded awareness into the moments that follow, or a longer meditation.

Trust

Trust in your own feelings and intuition is vital in a meditation practice, and in life. No one can tell you how you feel, and feeling with clarity takes the courage of your convictions. When you make time and space, anything can arise and when this is uncomfortable or something you struggle to stay with, breathing into your heart with trust and courage can help you hold space around it rather than hardening against it.

Positive visualization

Regular self-compassion practice (especially with touch) has been shown to both lower cortisol and raise the anti-stress hormone DHEA.[8,9] From an Eastern perspective, it nourishes our heart, the centre of compassionate energy. Positive visualization techniques use imagery to gather and focus this kindness inwards.

Practice: Learning to 'think with your heart'

This practice helps to recharge your batteries.

1. Stop and observe your emotional state, even name it if you can do so without getting caught up in the 'story'.

2. Name what is causing you stress, even write it down if it helps (this is good at night, to let go of thoughts or preoccupations that may interfere with sleep quality).

3. Focus on your heart area – put your right hand there.

4. Shift your attention to a happy, uplifting event, person or place in your life and spend a few minutes imagining it or them.

5. Bring something to mind that allows you to feel unconditional love or appreciation – for example, a child or a pet – and hold that feeling for as long as you need to, holding your hand over your heart or, if you need to bring your hand down, feeling the imprint of it there.

6. Note how you've been able to shift out of the downward spiral of negativity.

This practice offers refuge if you're feeling panicked, angry, guilty, fearful or anxious. It can be used as a nightly guided meditation if you have a busy brain, sleep issues and/or tend to give out more kindness to others than to yourself.

Asking questions

Curiosity is a fundamental part of mindfulness, and asking questions of ourselves helps bring us to the present and step back from trying to control the outcome. These questions help us to bring space to difficult moments.

Practice: Enquiry questions

Sit with your feet on the ground and close your eyes. Then take a deep breath and – if it feels right – put your hand on your heart. Now ask yourself the questions below. Take a few moments to *feel* (not think about) the answers, to allow you to discover what can cut through the noise when your head is spun by stress. You can play around with what you respond to best.

- What can I be grateful for right now? What can I let go of right now?

- Is the problem the situation, or was it my reaction to the situation? What can I let go of right now?

- What will happen if I don't get what I want right now? What can I let go of right now?

- Will this be important in five years' time? What can I let go of right now?

- What can I be grateful for right now?

The body scan

Many mindfulness courses start the home practice with a body scan, but it's a wonderful guide at any time, particularly when we feel too busy-minded to find it easy to 'be with ourselves'. Moving awareness through the body in a systematic way helps us experience sensations 'just as they are' – simply observing and letting go of evaluation, comment, analysis and comparison.[10]

This form of guided meditation is usually done lying down, to feel full body support, but you can sit on a chair if you're tending to fall asleep throughout. There are short and longer length recordings at www. charlottewattshealth.com and many others are available on the internet, particularly if you get used to just one voice or recording and the practice becomes automatic. Yoga nidra, the 'yoga of sleep', is a similar practice that often also invites you to set an intention (*sankalpa*) for your practice.

Body scans have been shown to reduce food cravings[11] and may help increase sensitivity to areas of the body that have decreased sensation through chronic stress or trauma.

Practice: The body scan

This simple version of the body scan, with affirmations, can be used to bring stillness to an agitated mind–body. Lying or sitting comfortably, move through the following places in your body with steady focus, saying all (or a few) of the phrases inwardly:

- My whole body is still; I'm occupying my whole body

- My hands are still; there is nothing to do

- My feet are still; there is nowhere to go

- My jaw is relaxing; there is nothing to tense against

- My face is softening; there is nothing to express

- My throat is soft; there is nothing to say

- My spine is moving with my breath; I am fluid

- My brain is still; there is no reaction needed

- My breath is softening; I feel peace

- My whole body is still; I can let go

Sensory mindfulness meditations

Our senses are how we meet and make sense of the world around us. They can be a route to mindfulness and either dulled or heightened as a result of trauma or long-term stress. Exploring their input consciously supports our attunement and trust of present experience.[12]

Touch

The reality and sensory feedback of your own touch can be physically and emotionally comforting. As mammals we respond to warmth and holding; hugs raise beta-endorphins and healing oxytocin (the hormone released when we feel love) and this is felt by your own touch as much as from someone else's.

In Eastern traditions the right hand signifies compassion and is laid over the heart to gather love there. The left hand signifies wisdom and can be placed on your belly to connect to intuition over busy head stuff. This can be used at any time we feel disconnected, lost or overwhelmed by emotional or physical sensations like food cravings. Walking meditation also uses touch from feet to ground to connect.

Taste

See the mindful eating exercise on page 93 and slow down during meals to let your brain register satisfaction from what you've eaten.

Sound

Include all the sounds around you as part of your practice; feeling your responses to noise without needing to react, judge or follow. You can also use the Insight app to make a singing bowl sound at intervals and follow the sound right to its very end vibrations. Gong baths, meditative music and nature sounds can give an agitated brain something to do, keeping the experience abstract rather than engaging the brain with lyrics. A chattering mind can be soothed by hearing words in chants (mantra) in a language it doesn't know and where the meaning doesn't distract.

Scent

Use aromatherapy oils or a favourite candle, flower or food smells to evoke feelings and notice mind–body responses.

Sight

Meditating with your eyes open means receiving visual information while remaining attuned to your internal landscape. You can even meditate upon an object, like a candle flame, with a soft, focused gaze (*drishti* in yoga).

Learning to see without grasping for more information can help soften our eyes and brains; this is important when our vision is so dominant and the many micro-movements we make with our eyes watching various screens is so tiring and stressful.

Find what works, then practise with consistency

Ten minutes daily of any type of meditative practice has the potential to reset our brain chemistry towards more adaptable and resilient 'grooves'. A smaller, consistent commitment to meditation or yoga has more benefit than the occasional half-hour and is more likely to result in a practice you feel is a vital part of your life.

Keeping a daily log of reflections can help you connect your practice to your life, but resist looking for it to 'fix' any aspect; let it simply help you be who you truly are. See the meditation recordings at www. charlottewattshealth.com

Help for your specific Stress Suit		
	Resistance to mindfulness	Best practice in-route
Stressed and Wired	Racing mind	Practising interceptions to stress; pausing in daily life to 'drop-in' and create space; walking meditation (see page 191)
Stressed and Tired	Can't be bothered	Sitting in silence to 'just be' – building up as feels right, e.g. 5, 10, 15, 20 minutes
Stressed and Cold	Just want to curl up in a ball	Body scan or yoga nidra under a blanket
Stressed and Bloated	Uncomfortable in posture	Mindfulness in daily life, especially when eating
Stressed and Sore	Staying still is challenging	Yoga practices or any other mindful movement
Stressed and Demotivated or Hormonal	Feeling negative thoughts or self-critical	Gratitude practice (page 161); positive visualization (page 193)

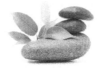

CHAPTER 16

Yoga as Awareness

*'The success of yoga does not lie in the ability to
perform postures, but in how it positively changes
the way we live our life and our relationships.'*
T.K.V. DESIKACHAR

The word *yoga* comes from the Sanskrit word for 'yoke' and translates
as *union*. This 'philosophy in action' is a system with many aspects, all
concerned with focus towards an integrated state. The physical practice
most associated with yoga today was a late addition to its meditative and
cleansing practices.

With its true emphasis for mind-body-spirit connection, the postures
(*asanas*) were added to help bring the body awareness and energy
balancing needed to 'still the mind' in preparation for meditation.
Practising the postures or any other aspect of yoga without mindfulness
within breath and body is simply just making shapes. In essence, we don't
actually *do* yoga, as union is something we can only *allow*.

Many people start a physical yoga practice because it does bring
muscular strength, tone, flexibility and endurance to the body, but most
continue it because of the sense of connection and contentment this brings
to the mind.[1,2] People with tight breathing, bodies and faces – as well as
difficulties 'letting go' – respond to the practice with great relief and steady
progress, unlocking physical and emotional stress held in the body.

Mindfulness is inherent within the practice and it helps us breathe through and accept any nature of these releases as we meet them on the way out. See the next chapter for morning and evening yoga practices.

> *'Yoga is not interested in solving anything, but
> rather revealing that which is already there.'*
> JIM TARRAN

STILLING THE MIND

In yoga, calm, long breaths as we move the body increase oxygenation, spare vital nutrients, reduce heart rate, relax muscles and reduce anxiety. This increases all-over communication throughout the body, including that between the brain, spinal cord and nerves.[3] The brain needs three times more oxygen than the rest of the body, so increasing this supply with conscious breathing can have immediately positive effects on mood, cognitive function and focus.

Patanjali's Yoga Sutra(s) – written c.2000BCE, and from which modern practices are derived – describe yoga as 'stilling the mind fluctuations'. We now know how this inherent wisdom is so effective – awareness of the body engages the right, visual-spatial hemisphere of the brain, thus dampening the left brain's internal commentary.

Yoga's ultimate aim is to attain *Samadhi* – utmost connection with the universe, a melding of individual consciousness with universal consciousness (whatever that means to you); that *nothingness* all meditative practices are moving towards. In practical terms this means cultivating connection between your breath, body and mind and revealing how you truly feel rather than how you *think* you feel.

Without this flow, being continually divided uses up a lot of energy and we can even push our bodies into idealized shapes and positions that neither suit nor serve them. *Ahimsa* or non-violence is the first *yama* (attitude) in yoga and is the self-compassion that allows us to treat our bodies as friends not enemies. The late guru B.K.S. Iyengar described this as 'effortless effort'.

Opening up

Many people say, 'I can't do yoga because I'm not flexible enough,' shying away from it because the initial releasing and lengthening of muscle can feel too intense. Your body is designed for flexibility as part of natural movement – to continually open up connective tissue – and it wants you to do that. Watch how an animal naturally stretches after a period of rest when connective tissue naturally contracts.

You might feel the same thing when you get out of bed or have been sitting for a while. Sitting on chairs is an endemic health problem – knees held at right angles for hours can make hamstrings seize up and contribute to tight hips, both common elements in lower back pain. If your body isn't used to stretching, it may resist at first, but you'll soon feel the joy of new habits and opening up.

What is flexibility?

Your body's mobility and agility depends on the expansion and contraction range of connective tissues around your joints. Age, a sedentary lifestyle and even over-exercise and repetitive movement can mean muscles contract around joints, limiting range of movement and leading to aches and pains.

Anything from 10–90 minutes a day spent stretching – through yoga, Pilates or dance stretching – can allow rehabilitation and help make exercise (particular running and cycling) a good stress rather than just driving your body into the ground. Promoting the stretching of key nerves that link joints to the brain can have profoundly de-stressing benefits in as little as 15 minutes, by promoting *vagal tone*, our ability to self-soothe via vagus nerve communication to the parasympathetic nervous system (PNS) (see page 38).[4]

A muscle stretch as a good stress is up to a safe and comfortable limit without any tension in other areas of the body to compensate. Allow long and spacious breathing to stay in any stretch; if we are literally 'gritting our teeth' to practise with short, shallow breaths, we've moved into strain and are engaging the sympathetic nervous system (SNS) (see page 38). This 'edge' continually changes, so modulate to how you feel in the moment, not what you've done before. There's no need to work right up to the edge; find it and then back away enough to be able to work with what Buddhists call *right effort*. That's not too much and not too little – a fine balance.

How yoga changes mind–body expressions

Learning to stay with yoga postures, breathing practices and meditation helps us to become more accepting and able to relax into what might previously have been perceived as discomfort or pain. What are simply strong sensations of release during a stretch, or change on a bigger scale, can cause us to react with sudden aversion, when our minds are slow to adapt.

Conditioning ourselves to breathe and relax with these messages to 'pay attention' helps us know, from true, gut feelings, what's really supportive and what's damaging. Then we can acclimatize to natural stress – exercise, intellectual challenges, being cold, feeling hunger – and become stronger.

As yoga reveals our true natures, we can often feel waves of the pain, sadness, anger, grief, needs, desires or even joys that we may not have been able to express. As we often mollify these feelings with food or other consumption, we can feel somewhat exposed when starting out. But we soon see this as part of an expansive journey. I often felt intense anger throughout classes when I first started yoga, which would make my teacher smile – we don't need to judge or even like what comes up!

Yoga is the perfect accompaniment to nutritional change. 15,000 long-term yoga practitioners were assessed by researchers and shown to put on lower-than-average weight over 10 years. The study didn't draw conclusions, but one theory is that yoga practice increases our ability to resist the discomfort of cravings as just another 'strong sensation'.[5]

Other studies have shown lowered body-fat levels, better appetite control and postural stability, body image and self-esteem and fewer food cravings.[6,7,8,9] It's likely these effects are linked to increased relaxing alpha brainwaves and anti-anxiety GABA (see page 53) and decreased levels of the stress hormone cortisol. Just one hour's yoga practice a week has been shown to help reduce stress and anxiety.[10,11,12]

Studies have also shown that yoga can help alleviate headaches, insomnia, sleep issues, depression, menstrual problems and lower back pain, and relieve high blood pressure and racing heart.[13,14] They've also shown that pain, and our reaction to it, decreases with yoga practice. Massage and yoga have been shown to elicit similar cortisol-lowering effects, with yoga described as 'self-massage' as your body rubs against itself and the floor. This and increased serotonin levels are believed to help shut down 'pain gateways'.

UNDERSTANDING YOUR BREATH

Breathing is the clearest signal of your body's state at any given time, as seen on page 39. Pulling air into the body and then releasing the waste product carbon dioxide involves large sets of muscles:

1. Diaphragmatic breathing – this uses the *primary breathing* muscles, the large upside-down-bowl-shaped diaphragm muscles at the bottom of your ribs. With an easy exchange of filling and emptying the lungs, the chest expands and the diaphragm moves downwards to inhale, rising back up as the chest drops to exhale. Lying down, this breathing can be seen as the belly rising and falling. It's the most energy-efficient, oxygenating breath and the least stressful to the muscular system.

2. Thoracic (chest) breathing – when we're stressed or the diaphragm can't move fully, our breath moves to the upper chest and shoulders; this is called *secondary breathing*. During the fight-or-flight response, this causes quicker, shallow breaths. Many people get stuck in this pattern, using up precious energy and creating tension in the neck and shoulders.

Research has shown that most people use just 25 per cent of their breathing capacity, tending to focus either into the top of the chest or just in the belly. Breath consciousness in yoga postures helps us feel and engage breath through the whole respiratory system and feel its currents right down to the pelvic floor and up into the head.

The nasal breath

When stressed, many of us breathe through our mouth rather than nose. Mouth-breathing is associated with poor posture (tipping head back to 'gulp' air) and tiring lack of oxygenation.[15] In yoga, all breathing, unless otherwise instructed, is through the nose, as yogis maintain that *prana* (life-force) from the breath only enters the body through the nose (and from nourishing food and sunlight).

From a scientific standpoint, nasal inhalations cool down the brain's frontal lobe, calming its activity and warming up air entering the lungs and body for easy oxygen uptake. They also help nitric oxide production, important for immune function and circulation. If you have nasal issues that make this difficult, look at the immune and inflammatory advice on pages 62–64.

Many yoga students are instructed that the ideal breath ratio is 1:2 inhalation to exhalation, but if your natural rhythm differs in any way, or the day's events have thrown you off-track, pushing a round peg into a square hole can actually create stress.[16] Reducing stress and improving posture help new breathing patterns evolve safely and organically.

In yoga, our relationship with the breath can be more consciously manipulative than in mindfulness, where we simply observe. That isn't to say we control forcefully, but recognize where it may be expressing habits and can introduce new possibilities, like a deep breath in through the nose and a sigh out to help accept strong sensations, or at the start of a practice.

A single breath involves:

* Inhalation – pulling the air into the body involves muscular contraction and creates energy, but it can create tension if done

with force. It's better to exhale fully, creating a vacuum into which the in-breath flows effortlessly, most efficiently into a body with least tension. Inhaling activates the energizing sympathetic nervous system, so we naturally enhance it when we want to feel motivated.

- Exhalation – at its best, this is simply letting go of the muscles that pulled in the in-breath. Stress can tend to make us inhale before the out-breath has completed, so allowing the exhalation to release right to its natural end-point helps its calming action through the parasympathetic nervous system. The exhalation can naturally lengthen as shoulders, chest and jaw relax more and we can use this to self-soothe.

A balance between the two helps find the happy relationship between stimulation and recovery that is the foundation of The De-Stress Effect.

Look at your face from the inside

A good first place to visit in any physical practice is our faces. Here we express so much – how we relay (or hide) our feelings to the world and one of the major ways we invite others to either approach or stay back. Within our meditative practices we can let go of communicating and the face can relax; this is a relief when many of us want to escape energy-rich human contact when tired.

To become aware of your face and jaw is to notice when you might be playing out habits. Frowning can become pretty set as your default expression and it sends a message to the brain that you must be facing a challenge and need to stay tense. Likewise, the stress response involves a clenching of the jaw to constrict muscles to the brain and increase blood flow for fast responses. These aren't needed in most of our lives and especially not in practices where we are inviting the body to relax.

A soft jaw and face – even a little smile – tell the body things must be okay and you can let go of vigilance, including that racing mind. Smiling in a strong yoga posture reassures your body there is no danger, even if it's a grimace! Every so often in practice and life, check that:

- You aren't clenching your jaw or gritting your teeth; you can even open the jaw wide to release around the ear socket and the base of the skull, settling to find space between your back teeth. You can stick out the tongue and waggle it around or swallow to help.

- You are soft across the forehead, around the temples and between the eyebrows; squeeze and release them if needed.

- You have soft eyes and a steady, soft gaze – these help counter the strain our eyes and brain receive from continually darting around to look at screens and take in more information than they should naturally process.

ALLOWING, NOT PUSHING

Stress is expressed in body tissues and we can feel physical, emotional and psychological effects as we release tensions pushed deep into areas like the hips, thighs, buttocks and lower back. These can rise upwards and may feel stuck in tight shoulders, neck, face and jaw. Stay aware of these areas and move and breathe in to them as needed.

To begin with, it's natural to resist and contract around intense feelings, like a stretch, release or craving, labelling them as 'pain'. As we stretch a muscle, it will contract first to protect itself while working out if it's safe to lengthen without damage. Easy breathing and a calm nervous system signal this safe release, but this can take up to several minutes for some muscles.

You can feel more resistance if you insist and push your will into the pose, but you'll make more progress by waiting and *allowing* – working with, not against your body. Using the breath to stay for deeper opening can change your perception to feeling intensity as *good* and use it as an alternative to giving in to a craving. This and the brain chemistry changes described earlier are how yoga has been shown to help with addictions.

Yoga philosophy is concerned with *transcending the ego*, so ambition in postures really misses the point. Letting go of conditioned behaviours to try hard and reach goals can cultivate the freedom to *just be* and ripple out into our lives. Holding rigidly can only be sustained for so long: finding the right channels with an open mind has so much more longevity and grace.

The Yoga Sutra *Stirra Sukha Asanam* – 'steadiness with ease in postures' – informs us that without ease, strength becomes brittle, and without focus, comfort lacks direction. Striking a balance between desire and contentment for where we are now is a continual internal conversation.

The balance you need, not the grooves you've created

In life as in yoga, we're often drawn to activities that reinforce habits rather than provide the new ones we need. In yoga these trodden paths are called *samskaras* and the practice is concerned with moving us out of these to reveal our true natures. It's recognized that people who tend towards overstimulation (*rajassic* or fiery) gravitate towards a more dynamic practice that feeds that, when they may need more quiet and calm. Those feeling fatigued (*tamassic* or dull) can fall into a purely restorative practice, when they might need to create more energy gradually.[17]

Between these opposite energies is the balanced, informed and sustaining state of *sattva*, where we can remain conscious enough to regulate to what we need, as we need it. As we tend to lurch between up and down in modern life, this can be a helpful viewpoint to find a middle path, even if it's challenging.

MOVEMENT EXPLORATIONS

Simply allowing ourselves to come to a state of presence and really feel 'What is true right now?' (many thanks to Tara Brach) sets the scene for movement. Coming directly to yoga postures from a stressed state can bring the gunk with us. Taking some time to identify where we're holding on means we have the opportunity to move it through and release, not embed, tension.

Stress in the belly

Coming right back to the gut stuff on page 12, connecting to how we feel at this primal, visceral location is the root to unlocking deeply held stress. With so much information about our wellbeing travelling from gut to brain, any postural shifts that support digestion may have implications back to 'still the mind'.

Physically our bellies are at the centre of our being, although our focus on thinking tends to make us believe that 'we exist' up in our heads. Losing belly connection can cut off our ability to listen and respond to what we really need. Digestive issues are a sure sign that gut messages aren't being heard and modern tendencies to hunch or slouch put pressure on the digestive organs with little opportunity for the stretching, compression and twisting they need.

Connecting to your gut and its expressions outwards can help you bring this awareness into daily life, during yoga poses or before meditation:

- Putting your hands on your belly can help you focus and breathe there, feeling the calming sensations of touch.

- Move feet and hands regularly to feed release back towards the belly – pointing and flexing, opening and closing, rotating joints or shaking out; these act as natural trauma release in many cultures.

- Tap your head and chest (or anywhere that feels right) lightly with fingertips to discharge tension from the central body.

Skull-sacrum polarity

Stagnation in the belly is also felt in the deep lymphatic tissues in the colon and around the groin. Opening up the inner thighs, hips and groin, as well as the belly, helps relieve compression in the colon and encourages lymphatic flow that helps elimination processes and immunity. The soothing vagal nerve signals body relaxation via nerves in the spine in the region of the adrenal glands and the belly.

Our ability to self-soothe comes with good balance between this sacral area and the nerves into the brain at the back of the skull (cranium), referred to as 'skull-sacrum polarity'. This is helped by cranio-sacral therapies, the spine undulations that follow, and letting yourself roll up and roll down through the belly between postures on different planes – for example, a standing forward bend to standing upright.

Releasing the jaw and checking habits of lifting the chin in everyday life and yoga postures can help open the base of the skull, which can be visualized as cooling moon, water or *yin* energy. Sitting hunched and then looking up (i.e. to look at a screen) can create compression at the top of the neck where it meets the skull. Tucking chin to throat lightly as you sit and stand can help retrain the length at the back of the neck, release tightness in the top of the back, flood ease down into the adrenals and belly and make space to open the chest.

Body-stress relieving movements

As well as the sequences in the next chapter, the movements below help you explore areas of the body where you feel stress held. Cortisol affects motor control so movements may seem jerky or uncoordinated to start, but the more we focus attention to move outwards from our belly centre, the more graceful movements of limbs become.

Then a stretch can feel more like a *reach*, not just pulling on joints, but moving more freely as our bodies were designed to, and where injury becomes a lot less likely. This also encourages fluidity, not just as a metaphor for moving with *flow*, but as stress makes bodily fluids more viscous and sticky, movement provides anti-ageing lubrication.

Moving our joints increases their oiling synovial fluid. Moving fluidly into the torso encourages 'slide and glide' in the viscera, where we can feel limited motion between organs that affects digestion and movement itself. Blood and lymphatic flow also help counter stress-related heart, immune and detoxification issues.

Sure and steady for fatigue

For those suffering burnout or fatigue, the simple motions in this chapter and poses 3, 12, 13 and 15 in the next chapter may feel enough, but do experiment; it's better to do some movement and need to recover afterwards than to be completely static. This is where muscle atrophies, we lose our natural imperative 'to move' and fluids pool and stagnate.

Walking regularly is a priority, even a little. At first the transition from this state may exhaust energy supplies and it's fine to feel you need a sleep or rest after. But by staying attuned, you can feel your way to building energy, strength and resilience intelligently.

Spine undulations

Exaggerating the natural movement of the spine as we breathe helps to unlock tension from the belly and sends a wave to move that through the whole mind–body. These movements have long been associated with improving digestion in many cultural practices, like belly dancing and kundalini yoga. Arching the back and opening the chest as the lungs fill to inhale, and rounding it as they empty on exhale, can be done in any plane and from many positions:

- See cat/cow pose page 216 as an example
- On a chair is good; at a desk for neck relief, and when tight hips make seated positions difficult
- Lying down with arms out to the side, as in the preparation for pose 12 on page 222. Support from the ground helps free shoulders in the process, as they don't need to be held up.
- In poses 1 and 10 (with hands on thighs) on pages 215 and 221.

The table position

As well as cat/cow pose (see page 216), coming onto all fours allows free movement of the spine with the safe feeling of being rooted to the ground. It also offers support for movement in the shoulders and hips that allows exploration of the 'fluid body' in the abdomen and viscera. Feeling your belly draw up to support your lower back here connects to core integrity for movement with awareness.

- Take your pelvis to one side and circle down with an exhalation towards child pose (see page 222) then draw up the other side as you inhale to complete a circle. Keep circling, drawing up through the belly as you rise and then change direction to feel the difference.

- Rotate the pelvis as if belly dancing, imagining the tip of the tailbone as a pencil, and draw large circles. Start in just the pelvis until looseness travels up the spine to include shoulders, neck and head – however feels right; then change direction.

- Lifting the right arm forward and left leg back. Lengthen between the two, with belly support and focusing the eyes forward and down; this can help encourage the balance and left-right brain integration that can suffer with chronic stress. Repeat on the other side.

Opening from the curling stress response

A withdrawal response to stress is to curl into a ball – the foetal position – where the vulnerable belly and heart are protected. This place can be a refuge to calm our nervous systems, either sitting or lying. Many yoga postures (such as 11 and 15 on pages 222 and 224) mimic this for us to gather in resources in a sequence or as a therapeutic aid.

This response (and sitting on chairs for long periods) tightens the psoas muscle, which lengthens for us to stand up; shortening through stress can be felt in tight thighs, lower back pain, belly constriction and breathing issues. The psoas is known to respond massively to emotions, so coaxing it open (for movements like lunging and back bends) needs self-compassion and deep de-stressing, as well as physical opening of the front body.

Constructive Rest Position (CRP) held for 15 minutes minimum allows full release of the psoas muscle, which can be felt as letting go down the thighs, into the belly and even into breath in the diaphragm. Here's how to do it:

- Lie with feet far enough away from your bottom to create a 90-degree angle between upper and lower legs, where you feel equal weight distributed between ball and heel of hip-wide feet. See more info at www.charlottewattshealth.com

If chronic stress makes opening the chest difficult, lying over a rolled towel or blanket at the bottom edge of the shoulder blades (bra strap line) daily with breath awareness helps entice opening at a rate your mind–body can feel is safe. Have legs bent to start, and you may be able to lengthen them out as you progress, if breathing doesn't tighten.

See also the positive visualization on page 193 to nourish the heart strength to let your body know it's safe to open up.

Sound and vibration

Adding sound into a yoga practice adds another healing dimension,[18] and you may find yourself sighing loudly at key points of release naturally. Go with it and feel free to express relief at any time:

- Soft throat and tongue – letting an 'ah' sound come out on exhalation opens the back of the throat and palate and creates releasing vibrations in the head; this can be useful when we're arriving at the beginning of a practice, or at any time we feel stressed. Any vowel sounds are useful and the mantra 'om', often referred to as the 'universal sound', resonates a deep connection with the Earth and so is often chanted three or more times at the beginning or end of a class.

- *Brahmari* or 'bee breath' creates a humming sound on the exhalation that encourages long, slow breath from the diaphragm and creates vibration in the upper torso and throat. The 'M' sound created vibrates into the cerebral cortex and has been shown to nourish the pituitary gland and regulate stress responses.[19] It's often practised seated, sealing the eyes and ears to direct sound inwards, but can also take the form of a hum on the out-breath in any pose, for example numbers 1, 10, 11 and 20 in the next chapter.

Namaste 'may the light in me honour the light in you'

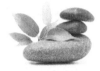

CHAPTER 17

The De-Stress Yoga Sequences

'When we bring our mind into our body, the body becomes mindful, and the mind becomes embodied.'
DONNA FARHI

The yoga sequences in this chapter are designed as a grounding for you to add to and modulate as you explore the poses – and the movement in the previous chapter – plus any you learn in a yoga class. You may also have physiotherapy exercises or beneficial Pilates moves that you can incorporate into the sequences. Discover what your body best responds to.

Yoga has always taken whatever forms work to reveal best health: if a movement is practised with embodiment and mindful intention, there is the yoga: *union.*

Each pose has a simple description to which you can add playful exploration. Sometimes we need to be more still; at other times we need to move stuff through – trust your inner voices. Feel the natural length of the pose for that day (it may be different each time you practise), connecting with your intuition rather than a specific breath count. Stay in the pose for as long as face, jaw and breath stay smooth; your body will tell you when you're 'cooked'.

Check with your doctor before starting any new movement regimen, especially if you have neck, head, shoulder, arm, wrist, back or knee issues or tend to headaches, dizziness, numbness, tingling or high blood pressure. Read the pose descriptions first to lessen confusion and then enjoy opening your body! Videos, pose variations, pictures and more sequences are at www.charlottewattshealth.com

If in doubt about the order of a sequence, you can safely add in a down-face dog (page 217) as a spine neutralizing or *bridging* pose at any time.

MORNING PRACTICE

This is a simple sequence focused on slowing down to sense all the nuances, flavours, subtle fluxes and messages from within, through the breath. When we speed up and rush past, these can blur and get missed – like a landscape rushing past from a train window. If you're used to a faster, stronger practice, this journey can feel unfamiliar and you may even feel resistance and the desire to 'do more'.

If you're feeling the effects of stress or even burnout, remember it's these desires to achieve that may get in the way of creating new grooves to live by. Our yoga practice helps us to notice these; wanting to rush through can also be a sign that you might tend to be focusing on the broader strokes and the end-point, rather than the subtle aspects of the journey. If you're used to a more vigorous practice, try this different approach with an open mind and you'll find it can complement other types.

'I trust my body to organize itself as it knows how to do.'

We can feel naturally tight in the morning, so work with some energy to spare, and space for muscles to wake up gradually, *inviting* your body into the practice. Aim to complete the morning sequence at least three to four times a week, taking the time that feels right for your body. There is no set time for each pose – that can get in the way of your felt sense. The whole sequence is around 15–25 minutes.

Set a soothing alarm (or use the Insight app) for at least one or two minutes before you need to stop, for time to lie in Savasana (corpse pose) at the end of the sequence and make a smooth transition into your day. Do not skip Savasana – it's crucial for assimilating the effects of your practice deep into your tissues.

Pose 1: Siddhasana (Adept's pose, loose version)

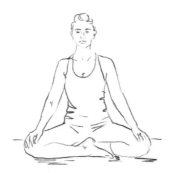

- Sitting on at least one block or cushion to allow lifting through the front spine and from the back of the pelvis, take each buttock out and back to sit up from the sitting bones.

- Allow the spine to rise on the inhalation and shoulders to release as you exhale.

- Allow the legs to drop down and knees to soften with each out-breath – to feel the lower body rooting to the Earth allows the spine to grow to the sky.

Explorations

- Hands down onto the thighs is a more grounding action, often helpful for an agitated brain. The *mudra* (gesture or energy seal) often seen in meditation photos – palms up, index finger and thumb touching – is *jnana mudra*, representing wisdom and receptivity and a sensory meditative focus.

- Circling the whole spine (like an upside-down pendulum) in both directions creates lubrication of the hip joints. Move the chest in circles to feel the motion into the hips, keeping the shoulders soft.

- Any number of spine, back, shoulder and neck loosening practices can be done from this pose. Try the spine undulations on page 210. Rolling the shoulders and rotating the neck from side to side are just a few more – feel free to explore.

Pose 2: Parivrtta Siddhasana (twist variation)

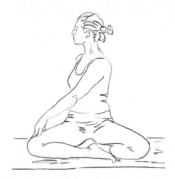

- Still sitting on your block or cushion, feel the crown of the head lift up directly over the sitting bones, inhale height through the spine to limit compression and twist to the right on the exhalation.
- Turn from the belly and then the chest, not just the neck. Repeat other side.

Exploration
- Counter-rotating the neck in twists can encourage lymphatic drainage via the upper chest that helps immune and detoxification function. Turn the head towards the front shoulder and even exhale to there, inhale back and follow this neck movement as feels good, before holding to the front.

Pose 3: Marjaryasana/Bitilasana (cat/cow pose)

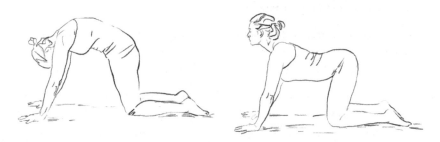

- From all fours, hands below the shoulders and knees under hips, with an exhalation, lift the spine up, dropping the head. With an inhalation, drop the spine between shoulders and hips, lengthening through the whole neck, instead of just lifting the chin.

- Let movement follow each breath to the end.
- Continue until shoulders and spine fully loosen into this 'moving meditation', feeling support and uplift from the ground.

Explorations
- See other loosening possibilities from all fours on pages 210–11.

Pose 4: Adho Mukha Svanasana (down-face dog)

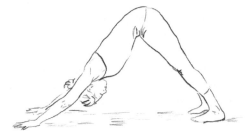

- From all fours, hands spread and middle fingers parallel, exhale as you lift the bottom to the ceiling, heels up, legs bent to start.
- Push back and up from the base of the index fingers (the 'brains of the hands') to lengthen through the shoulders and lift the tailbone.
- Rather than forcing the heels down, draw up the knees and allow the heels to move back and down as you push back from the palms to draw the top of the thighs back and open the back of the legs.
- Stay as long as your breath can flow, then walk your feet towards your hands to Uttanasana (pose 5) with bent legs.

Explorations
- Rather than just pedalling the legs to open the hamstrings, also explore moving out of the forward-back plane. Figure-of-eight sideways motions through hips and shoulders create a more fluid relationship with the pose.

Therapeutic help: if you have wrist issues in this pose, coming to the elbows is an option, but it may be too intense for those with tight shoulders. An alternative is to place the whole palms on blocks, allowing the fingers to drop to relieve the wrist angle.

Pose 5: Uttanasana (intense stretch pose)

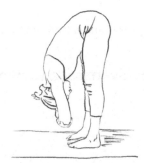

- With feet hip-width apart, outer edges parallel, hold elbows and hang from the hips, bending the knees if you need to, or feel any pull on the lower back.

- Explore drawing up through the knees and dropping into front heels to lift sitting bones to the sky. Be mindful not to lock the lower back.

- Bend legs and roll up the spine to standing on an in-breath.

Explorations

- Awaken the feet from their 'brain' – the ball of the big toe – by lifting and spreading your toes every so often, to lift up through the inner legs.

- Simply hanging the arms and moving the head in a 'yes' and 'no' motion can help release neck and shoulders.

- A softer version can be like a 'standing child pose' (see pose 11) with torso dropping down onto thighs with bent legs; you roll up to standing and back down again several times to ground down through the feet.

Pose 6: Tadasana (mountain pose)

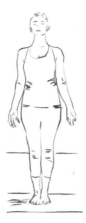

- Stand, feet together or apart, as feels right, feet open and supportive yet soft to feel the whole body rise up from the floor to the crown of the head.

- Let your breath create trust in your body's ability to organize best posture and gather into the midline for energy upwards. Let go of the need 'to do' or fix and simply stand and breathe.

*'I feel the ground and support of the Earth, with
space to move freely from firm roots.'*

Explorations

- Awaken feet as in Uttanasana, drawing up insteps, then inner thighs to support spine lift from the pelvic floor without constriction.

- Close your eyes and feel feet rooted into the Earth to allow you to sway freely and regain balance continually.

- Open feet into a wider stance, with knees slightly bent, and swing arms around like heavy weights on a rope for a rhythmic, twisting motion.

Therapeutic help: although this illustration shows the 'traditional' pose with feet together, directly hip-width apart is more comfortable and stable for many – especially women who have given birth and those with lower back issues.

Pose 7: Vrksasana (tree pose)

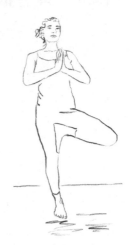

- From Tadasana, pose 6, find a steady focus point and slowly move the weight onto the right foot. Lift the left foot and place onto the inner thigh or inner calf. Bring your hands into prayer position at the heart or lifting to the sky if you feel steady.

- Press the foot into the leg and vice versa, to gather energy in and rise up. Breathe into your focus point to balance.

- Bring the foot down to meet the other, settling in Tadasana before moving to the other side.

Therapeutic help: if you have difficulty balancing, rather than reaching for a wall, keep the tip of the big toe just touching the ground for a sense of safety. Then your nervous system can start to rebuild communication between the visual system (eyes), vestibular system (ears) and proprioception (the body's sense of where it is in space), which is interrupted by stress and needed for balance.

Pose 8: Uttanasana

As before (see page 218), from standing hip-width apart:

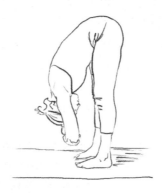

Pose 9: Adho Mukha Svanasana

As before (see page 217).

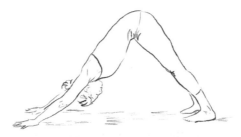

Pose 10: Vajrasana (diamond pose)

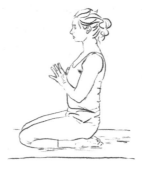

- Sitting with bottom on the heels (with blocks between if needed), drop down top of thighs and feel the spine lift up through its natural curves from the back of the skull.

- Bring the hands together into the heart for a point of breath focus.

- If difficult for your knees, come to all fours.

Explorations

- As with pose 1, this is a good starting position for any upper body movement.

Therapeutic help: tucking the toes under and sitting back creates 'interesting' sensations to breathe with; it also wakes up the feet and opens them up for best support when standing. Interlinking your fingers and turning palms up to the sky with arms raised above your head opens out the finger joints and encourages lymphatic flow. Activating hands and feet helps awaken the whole body and encourages staying present.

Pose 11: Balasana (child pose)

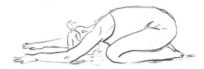

- From Vajrasana bring the big toes together, open the knees and walk your hands forwards, allowing time to release the lower back and eventually bring the hairline to the floor or onto one or two blocks.

- Breathe into the tops of the thighs and .back of the pelvis to release them down. Let the elbows drop to the ground to release the shoulders.

- Walk the hands back towards the knees, rolling up through the belly to come up head last.

Explorations
- You can make this more dynamic by stretching the arms out and tucking the toes under to give the push through the hands and feet to lengthen the spine.

- Rolling from side to side in Balasana loosens the sides of the body.

Pose 12: Supta Matsyendrasana (supine lord of the fishes pose)

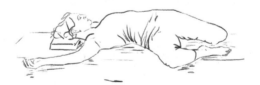

- Lie with legs bent, aligning outer edges of the feet with edges of the mat.

- Open your arms out to a wide position, elbows comfortably bent to where your wrists can drop (if they lift this may be shoulder tightness), often wider than 90 degrees.

- Inhale and then, on the exhalation, allow the knees to drop to the right side, rolling onto the sides of the feet. Let gravity take the weight of the legs down, release any gripping in the knees. Inhale back to centre, then exhale down to the left.

Explorations

- This can be practised as a flowing motion for loosening, dropping legs to the side as you exhale, to centre on inhale, and then move from side to side – aka 'windscreen wipers'.

- You can let the head move in the opposite direction to the legs, as feels comfortable, for a neck counter-rotation.

- On holding the side position, you can deepen it by lifting the bottom foot and positioning it on the outside of the top thigh; breathe into this 'rooting weight' to feel gravity and allow you to breathe opening into the spine from this point.

Therapeutic help: 'windscreen wipers' are a good start to a practice when stress has tightened your lower back. Moving from the floor allows easy motion that relieves core muscle tension that can interfere with natural back support.

Pose 13: Setu Bandha Sarvangasana (bridge pose)

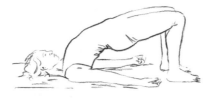

- Remove any head support and tuck the chin lightly to the throat. Place feet comfortably close to the buttocks, hip-width apart or wider if your lower back needs.

- With hands palm-up by the hips, inhale and lift the pelvis off the floor one vertebra at a time. Keep rooted in the feet, (especially the base of the big toe), roll the thighs in, flatten the belly and lift the heart.

- Stay as long as you can lift your chest with easy breath and soft face. Roll the spine down and rest until the back muscles settle.

Explorations
- This can be practised as a loosening motion at the beginning of a practice – rolling up on an inhale, down on an exhale and repeating. Arms can also be lifted up and over the head as the pelvis lifts, back down with the out-breath as it descends.

Pose 14: Supta Matsyendrasana

As before (see page 222); to release lower back; feel free to then move about, however feels right.

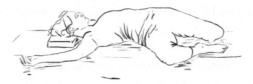

Pose 15: Apanasana (wind-relieving pose)

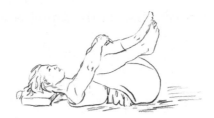

- Start from lying with soles of the feet on the floor, legs bent, head supported if shoulders are tight.
- Draw the knees up into the chest, looping the arms around the shins or the back of the thighs. Allow the knees to drop open and the weight of the legs to start deepening the hips over time. Place feet on the ground before moving to Savasana.

Therapeutic help: roll across the pelvis, spine and shoulder blades for a massaging effect.

Pose 16: Savasana (corpse pose)

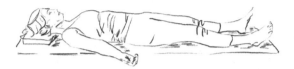

- Lie with your head on a low lift if your head tips back when you lie down. With arms comfortably away from the body, lift each shoulder blade down the body to open the chest. Stay for two to three minutes minimum – 10 minutes is optimal when you have enough time.

- Bend your legs and roll onto your side, lie for a few breaths before making a smooth transition into your day.

Focus guides

The following can help to hold your attention in Savasana or as simple meditation guides at any time:

'I'm breathing in calm; I'm breathing out space.'

- Visualize the exhalation making space by releasing stagnant energy, tension and anything that doesn't serve you; then the inhalation simply rushes in naturally to fill your whole body with fresh, new energy.

- Breathe into your belly and out to the whole of your body to soften your outer shell; this encourages us to meet the world with the awareness that promotes empathy and intuitive self-protection, rather than with a defensive, hard shell.

- Watch the inhalation rise up from the end of your toes to the crown of your head and the exhalation sweep out tensions ready to leave out and beyond your toes, feeling your breath like a tide.

Morning practice in full

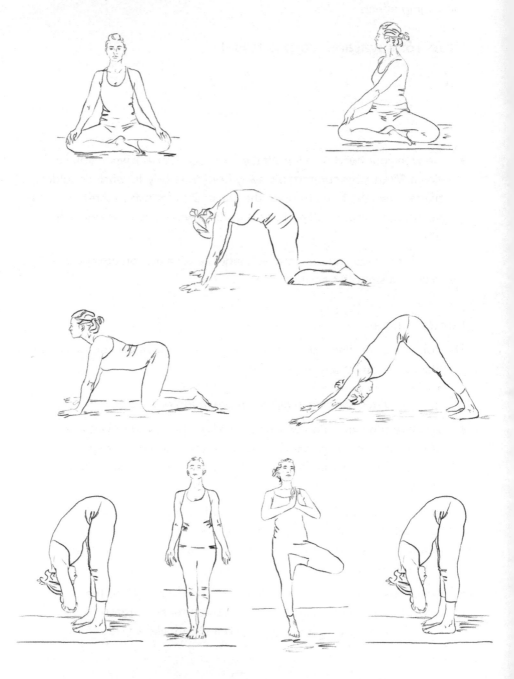

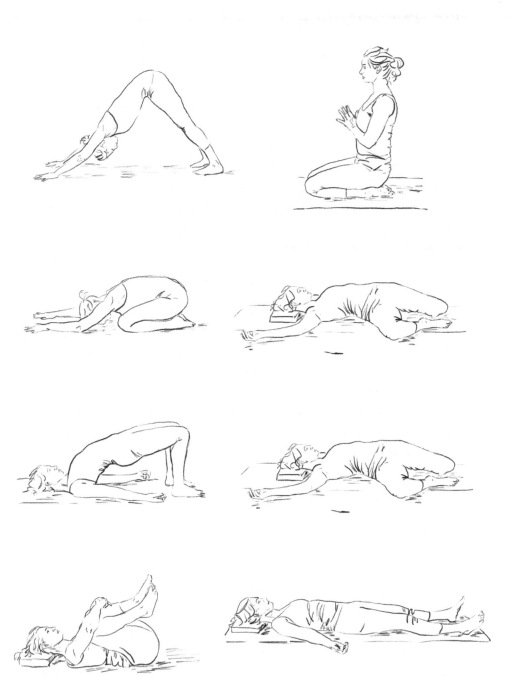

EVENING PRACTICE

Our bodies can be more open in the evening than in the morning, after daily movement, so flexibility comes more easily, helping us wind down and release the day – although you may find you need to move some stresses through first with stronger poses, like the Morning Practice.

You'll see some poses here described as 'restorative'. This is a specific practice where the body is positioned so it has to exert no muscular force to relax fully into a mindful, meditative state. If there's any pain or discomfort, adjust to relieve it, but also give yourself a chance to settle in with the breath and see how your body responds. You can stay in restorative poses for a while, feeling the time that's right for you. Move gently between poses with soft eyes and brain.

'I surrender and yield into what I need.'

If you need something simple or short that you can fully surrender into, *Evening Priority poses* are highlighted with an asterisk (*). One or two of these can fully relax mind–body to take you towards sleep. Apanasana, followed by Jathara Parivartanasana and then Savasana is a simple and effective practice.

You can do the evening practice as often as you like, nightly if suits. At least three to four times weekly will help establish your body's pre-sleep calming signals.

Pose 17: Apanasana

As morning practice (see page 224).

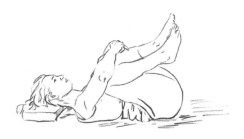

Pose 18: Adho Mukha Svanasana

As morning practice (see page 217).

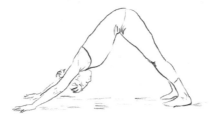

Pose 19: Balasana

As morning practice (see page 222), restorative version.

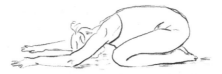

- To stay longer in child pose, you can support the head and torso with a bolster or a couple of pillows, turning the head to face each side for an equal amount of time.

Pose 20: Siddhasana forward bend (restorative variation to chair)

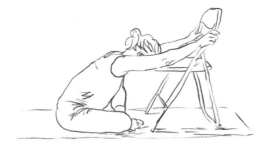

- Facing a chair in Siddhasana (pose 1 from morning practice), lengthen the spine by reaching to the back or sides of the chair, eventually resting the forehead on the chair seat (with optional cushions).

- Arms can be extended or folded on the seat – move the chair if you need to and find a position where the neck is long and comfortable.

- Drop into the sitting bones to safely extend the back muscles. Sit up slowly, change the cross of the legs and repeat.

Pose 21: Jathara Parivartanasana* (revolved abdomen pose, restorative version

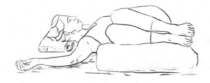

- Have a bolster or stack of towels (your 'lift') by your right ribs, skull supported if needed. Open your arms out with elbows comfortably bent.

- With knees into the chest, inhale to lift the pelvis and exhale to drop the legs onto the support. Stay to release, broaden collarbones and allow the left shoulder to drop without pushing.

- Inhale legs to centre, exhale to floor; rest and repeat other side.

Therapeutic help: supine (lying) twists provide spinal support to deepen with least compression between vertebrae.

Pose 22: Supta Baddha Konasana* (supine bound angle pose, restorative)

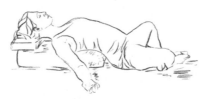

- Move your 'lift' lengthways, have cushion or block at the far end for your head. Sit with soles of the feet together where your hips feel comfortable.

- Lie over your lift, lengthening your lower back to avoid compression there; with neck comfortable, arms as in Savasana.

- Support outer thighs equally with cushions if any pulling there. To come out, press into the floor with the hands and come up in one breath.

Pose 23: Viparita Karani* (waterfall practice, restorative)

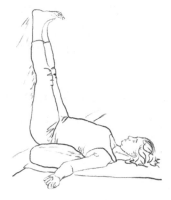

- Position your lift parallel and a couple of inches away from a wall. Sit on the end of your lift, lower hip close to the wall and swing legs up. Shimmy your lower back fully onto the lift, so the pelvis is supported but not digging into the waist; arms to the side or over your head. For tight hamstrings, move the lift further away from the wall.

- To come out, roll off your lift with one breath, lying on your side before coming up.

Therapeutic help: supported or restorative inversions allow a long, calming stay to cool and soothe an agitated brain. This pose creates cooling space at the base of the skull to release tension there and nourish the blood-brain barrier. This area relates to the optic nerve, often overstimulated by screen information.

Opening the legs wide allows gravity to drop into the pelvic organs. As a sudden tightening of the pelvic floor is an immediate stress response, we often have difficulty releasing in these areas, and it can even lead to stagnation as in constipation.

Pose 24: Savasana*

As morning practice (see page 225), always restorative.

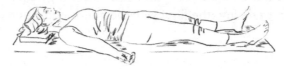

Option to support the legs over a bolster or rolled blanket, place an eye pillow or scarf over your eyes to cut out the light and cover yourself with a blanket to feel cocooned. This sense withdrawal (*pratyahara*) is an important part of a yoga practice and can be a safe refuge from the stimulation of the day.

Therapeutic help: if you're very tired, doing just this pose is a beneficial and complete practice: give in to it! You can also do body scans or an audio yoga nidra (see page 160).

Evening practice in full

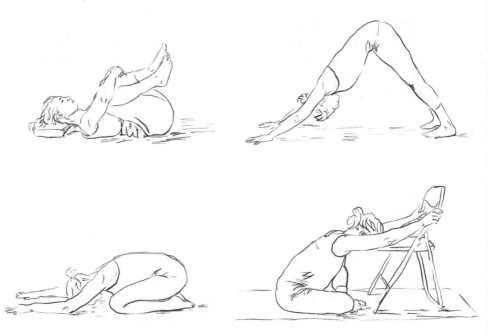

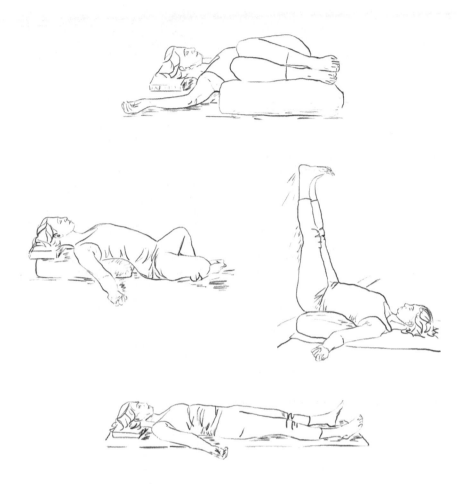

BLENDING HOME PRACTICE AND CLASSES

Yoga classes provide the anatomical and instructional attention crucial for safe practice – if you can't manage a weekly class even a few personal sessions or regular workshops can help. Videos can offer real instruction but can't provide personal adjustment or advice. Home practice ultimately means the chance to be more intuitive and respond to what you need. It's best supported by classes with a teacher you trust and who encourages you to feel and listen to your body. A class should leave you feeling both energized and calm, not hyped up.

Yoga practice by Stress Suit		
	You may find that you...	Your focus
Stressed and Wired	feel frustrated at not being able to get into that stronger/harder/bendier position	'Flexibility envy' is a term used by yoga teachers to help us notice ambition and ego creeping in. More force means more tension and less likelihood of a deep stretch, so let go into the breath.
Stressed and Tired	want to just lie down and drift off	Yes, restorative positions do restore, but do them alongside more energizing poses like adrenal-supporting twists to encourage oxygenation to help reduce fatigue.
Stressed and Cold	feel pain, tingling, numbness or pins and needles when you practise	Opening the throat and increasing circulation around the upper chest and thyroid is beneficial. Breathe into sensations arising as circulation improves.
Stressed and Bloated	find it difficult to connect to belly breathing and postural support as your abdomen tends to swell	Twists, with an emphasis on squeezing viscera, give intestines and bowel a massage to improve elimination. Breathe lying down to allow the diaphragm to move and abdominal contents to relax.
Stressed and Sore	feel pain or tightness in joints when you move into postures	Check that all postures are safe for you with a doctor or osteopath. Pain that changes when you move tends to be structural, but continual pain whatever your position is often more inflammatory.
Stressed and Demotivated	intend to but ultimately can't be bothered to start a yoga practice	Start small: even five minutes of cat/cow, down-face dog, child pose, one of the floor twists and then Savasana will have positive effects and motivate you more.
Stressed and Hormonal	feel vast differences in your postures at different times of the month	Supta Baddha Konasana is the ultimate PMS and hormonal pose, bringing circulation and connection to the groin area.

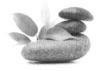

CHAPTER 18

The New Mind–body Movement

*'Don't get set into one form, adapt it and build
your own, and let it grow, be like water.'*
BRUCE LEE

If you were able to ask one of your hunter-gatherer ancestors to undertake some of today's exercise regimes, he'd look at you as if you'd just dropped your loincloth. Too many long, drawn-out periods of intense running, or repetitive movements on machines would exhaust his energy, perhaps injure him and put so much stress on his system that there would be no vitality for life's duties, like finding dinner or running away from predators set on making his family *their* next meal.

Today we don't have such problems and physical threats are a rarity in our cushioned lives. But emotional and psychological ones aren't – they don't get resolved as easily and they come with the same biological responses.

NATURAL CORTISOL RELIEF

In a stressful life, exercise is essential to provide the activity needed to burn off hormones that flood our systems during the 'fight or flight' response. The insulin, adrenaline and cortisol mobilized when you're under stress will promote fat storage if you sit at your desk stewing with anxiety and raised glucose. By using the energy that stress generates, physical activity can reduce its physiological impact on your body and make you feel better, faster – even if what's causing your stress is still there.

Exercise has been shown to lower levels of circulating cortisol naturally, be comparable – and in some cases better – for your mood than anti-depressants,[1] increase emotional resilience[2] and raise levels of immune-supporting probiotic gut bacteria. Exercise increases your metabolic rate, lessening the likelihood of stress contributing to excess fat around your belly.

The aim of The De-Stress Effect is to move away from hard, long workouts once or twice a week and think more in terms of significantly increasing the amount of activity in your daily life. Short, non-exhaustive movement sessions of varying intensity (as general activity and structured exercise) have more benefit than fewer long, energy-draining ones that most people only have the resources to do once or twice a week.

An emotional and physical fix

Today's most enlightened fitness experts are labelling notions of gruelling 'no-pain, no-gain' exercise as dated because they leave us leaner in the short term but stressed and exhausted in the long term, so we're more likely to lay down fat than build muscle. For those who don't tend to weight gain, excess amounts of the stress hormone cortisol can lead to muscle wasting and that sinewy, starved look that's often a telltale sign of an over-exercised, overstressed and possibly undernourished and under-hydrated body.

Studies are now showing that the strong correlation between physical activity and psychological wellbeing is most pronounced with low to moderate physical activity. One study of 12,018 people found that those who made physical activity part of their leisure time were less prone to stress and feelings of dissatisfaction.[3]

All this goes beyond simple endorphin rushes to a deeper sense of wellbeing and comfort in your own skin. Unless exercise is helping you alleviate negative emotions, not creating them by stressing or exhausting your body, it won't work long term and you won't keep it up. And the best news? What makes you feel good will probably make you look good too.

The best of good stressors

Remember the good stressors that make you stronger (see pages 46–47)? Exercise tops that list because the challenge it offers cardiovascular, hormonal, muscular and skeletal systems makes them come back stronger. All the benefits we know of exercise – increased metabolism and muscle tone, less tension and anxiety, more energy and glowing skin – are signs of the body's adaptation to these demands.

Your body has a natural day-to-day equilibrium, the biological point at which it feels and behaves its best. Too much ongoing, chronic stress can reset this ideal balance at a heightened rate, so the body expects more stress; over-exercise has a similar effect. But the right kind of exercise, in regular bouts and alternated with regular periods of deep rest, challenges that equilibrium in a positive way.

The heart rate goes up, muscle temperature and oxygen consumption rise but then get the chance to come down. Done regularly over time, this informs your body to get stronger and more efficient in response.

Naturally, our body's function peaks in the mid-thirties. From then on, basic fitness and aerobic capacity, as well as mobility, flexibility and strength, reduce. Ironically, this is often the time in our lives when psycho-social stress may be at its worst and we need these physical qualities most. By provoking an adaption response to the regular stress of exercise we can slow that progression down and build stress-coping resources, with the welcome by-product of a slim, toned, calm and comfortable body.

WE EVOLVED TO MOVE – PRIMAL FITNESS

Some 2.4 million years ago, humans evolved into the *Homo sapiens* species we are today, and for the majority of that time – about 84,000 generations – we lived as hunter-gatherers. Survival within that lifestyle required plenty of necessary movement and calorie-burning from finding food and water, social interaction, escaping from predators, building homes, washing clothes and carrying babies.

Though millions of years have passed since then, our bodies and their capabilities have remained genetically and physically the same – but our lifestyles have changed beyond recognition. Hunter-gatherers existed until about 10,000 years ago, which in evolutionary terms isn't long, and their lifestyles meant they weighed an average of 14kg (30lbs) less than we do today, while expending about 400–600 calories more every day. This was mostly in the pursuit of food and precious calories, cultivating a respect for food eaten.

Today we have ready-made food, people to build our homes, technology to do our work and, for most of us, daily toil involves more brain than body; we exercise only our fingers at our keyboard while the rest of our body sits and sits and sits (as I am indeed doing right now). In fact, according to a report in the *International Journal of Sports Medicine*, the energy expenditure of a typical Westerner is about 38 per cent that of our hunter-gatherer ancestors.[4] The bottom line is this: our bodies *love to move*. We evolved to move in many and varied ways.

If you think you hate exercise, it's probably because you've got used to a level of inactivity that means the beginning of movement comes with a certain level of discomfort. Mindfulness within our lives and extended into our movement patterns allows us to create new perceptions of unfamiliar feelings we might label as pain, so that we can feel these as good stress.

Discomfort along the way can be release of habitual tension and reorganization of postural and muscular alignment, to allow you to learn to love movement. Start slowly and give yourself time to listen to your body as you build up strength and the ability to move and use oxygen efficiently. You'll go through highs and lows, but keep at it and you'll soon feel the benefits of exercise, which include increased wellbeing and calm and less tension.[5]

Spontaneous activity

A crucial component of De-Stress fitness is 'spontaneous' or 'background' activity. Also known as 'incidental' exercise, it's simply about moving more in the context of your day – wherever you are, whenever you can. This isn't about heading off to the gym twice a week, but about moving around more often and increasing the amount of natural daily activity.[6]

One of the downsides to the rise of gym culture is that, having worked out, people may think being sedentary the rest of the time is okay. For our bodies, this sudden shift from 0–100 miles an hour is a pretty stressful jolt, especially when muscles have tensed and fluids settled through stress and lack of movement. We need to move regularly; no movement for more than an hour is basically sedentary and the metabolism starts to slow down.

Walking

Walking is our most natural form of exercise. It clears the mind, improves mood, has been shown to decrease cravings[7] and doesn't cost us energy or stress out the joints and muscles in the way that running does. We evolved to walk or lightly jog and can keep up this level of endurance for a very long time. When humans run, their energy costs are up to twice those of other mammals.

Our lymphatic systems rely on the particular movement that walking produces for immunity and detoxification. Ten thousand steps (around 3km/2 miles) a day is a basic requirement for this function, and for muscle health and fluidity in joints and around organs. We can soon see symptoms like dull skin, stiffness, sluggish digestion and brain fog when we stop moving.

Walking also produces a figure-of-eight movement through the spine, with its middle creating a supportive massage across the adrenal gland area. This gives a de-stressing rhythmic motion through our lower back, abdominal muscles and organs: the opposite to the rigidity caused by sitting in one position on a chair hour after hour.

This rhythm is halted into a purely forward motion when we break into a run, so a walk-run – walking for a minute, jogging for a minute – can create a medley of benefits, with time to recover between runs. You can vary this according to the day's energy to work with not what your stress-driven mind can push you to do, but what your body truly needs on any given day or week: movement without exhaustion.

If regular walking isn't a habit for you, get a pedometer and aim to clock up between 10,000 and 12,500 steps a day about five or six times a week.[8] Every step counts, even walking to the kitchen to make a drink. Roughly speaking, 5,000 steps is about half an hour's walking. Both regular short bursts (i.e. going to a toilet further away from your desk) and more dedicated exercise sessions have benefits, but the more you can walk on uneven terrain (and include hills), the more your musculoskeletal system benefits from the continual adaptation needed and the more meditative the movement becomes, as you need to focus on foot positioning.

Taking the stairs

Research published in the *British Journal of Sports Medicine* found that women who ran up and down the stairs at work for two minutes at a time, five times a day, boosted their fitness over an eight-week period.[9] Most of us are time-poor, but if you get up and move around every hour or so by running up a couple of flights of stairs, you're keeping your metabolism more lively than if you were sitting down for four hours straight.

Here are some other spontaneous activities to try:

- carrying shopping bags home – evenly distribute the weight over both arms
- having sex (a great de-stressor)
- gardening
- cycling to and from work
- stroller-walking
- vigorous housework
- carrying and chasing after a baby
- doing DIY
- dancing

FIT TO REST

Hunter-gatherers had a practical reason for being fit: so they could feed their families and, well, survive. That is why they would have had a widely varied system of movement and would have alternated difficult days with less demanding ones wherever possible, for full cell renewal and tissue repair.[10,11] This would have reduced the likelihood of crippling injuries that could be fatal in their environment.

In fact, while we know that physical exercise has many protective health benefits, including lowering our blood pressure and risk of heart disease, there is accumulating evidence showing that extreme physical activities over a prolonged period may be detrimental to health.[12] The pattern of exercise that we're genetically best suited to is a variety of activities performed intermittently and with different levels of intensity – not always high – and adequate rest in between to ensure complete bodily and muscle recovery between exertions.

When an athlete trains over a year-long period, they periodize their programme to have short, long, interval and variable training days mixed with rest or active recovery days. But lay people and the 'recreational elite' (those who do a triathlon or marathon) are often the ones who get injured or burned out because they train too hard, too soon: believing the training should match the length and intensity of the race.

It isn't uncommon to see those with adrenal fatigue take on a marathon just before they crash. Through habits of pushing themselves too hard, the imperative to achieve overrides any mindful connection to listen and take notice when their bodies are telling them they are tired. This is treating the body as if it were an enemy not a friend – and the compassionate (and effective) attitude is to rest when needed.

Alternate your workouts

Muscles and connective tissues need time to adapt to the mini-stressors that strength exercise puts on them, and they can't do this without rest. Alternating hard workouts with easy ones and having plenty of rest days actually produces better long-term fitness and has a far greater effect on your mood.

Vary it

There is no one-size-fits-all form of fitness – fully de-stressing movement needs to get you active in lots of different ways that suit you. In this way exercise becomes a natural part of your everyday life instead of yet another thing on your to-do list or reason to feel guilty. Remember that this is what suits your body, not your ambition; check you're listening to how you feel, not think. Don't feel the need to cram all the elements into any given week.

GET TOGETHER

Studies have shown that people get a boost in mood when they have the chance to socialize with friends, family and colleagues.[13] Ironically, those of us who are more introverted may benefit most from such interaction. 'Social Setting Exercise' is any activity involving more than one person – like squash, badminton, cricket, rounders, etc. These help us connect with other people, have fun and engage in some healthy competition.

We are pack animals and cohesion of the tribe is key to survival, so our brains reward these behaviours with a shot of the happy chemical dopamine. Our large brains evolved through the cooperation needed for hunting so this can feel right on a primal level and the reason many feel great de-stressing effects from games that employ this shared acuity of our physical beings and senses. This shifts us into a more attuned and present place, which provides rest from the overstimulated mental states and heightened stress hormones a working day can produce.

The following are some Social Setting Exercise forms that incorporate proven emotional as well as physical wellbeing benefits, raising feel-good beta-endorphins and the anti-stress hormone DHEA:

Dancing

For hunter-gatherers, dancing would have been performed as part of rituals and cultural celebrations and would have burned a massive 500 calories an hour. More importantly, we know dancing not only improves fitness, it also reduces stress. In fact, it's also been shown to improve memory, mood and cognitive (brain) functioning in the elderly and to help lower blood pressure.[14] Tribal-style dancing, like shamanic and 5 Rhythms, recreates the group healing of free expression through our bodies that is a traditional part of all ancient cultures.

Having sex

Large studies have found that people who have sex regularly report a host of health benefits, including raised immune function and lower mortality and risk of heart disease. It's often the last thing we feel like doing when we're stressed, but keeping that connection alive in a relationship does wonders for our sense of wellbeing and happiness; even a 'quickie' can make us feel better. Sex stimulates our bodies to produce hormones called prolactin and oxytocin, which are associated with improvements in mood and psychological bonding.[15,16] A sensual connection with a partner can enliven the senses and free mind habits.

Nature hikes

The challenging and beautiful terrain you negotiate on a hike in the countryside provides the perfect De-Stress Social Setting Exercise. A study in 2008 of groups hiking along the Appalachian Trail in the USA reported multiple benefits including physical challenge, self-fulfilment, warm relationships with others, fun and enjoyment of life and, of course, great exercise.[17]

Hikes can also be done silently (or part of the way), to practice mindfulness with others. Removing the habit of experiencing what we see and feel as we walk, through discussion and comment, means we truly get to feel the landscape in all its glory. It's easy to miss it if we're chatting about the mortgage or our job. If these things are causing you stress, appreciating the beauty of where you are right now can allow you to shift to a place of gratitude.

Negative ions: positive vibes from outdoor exercise

Some researchers believe that the reason we feel so good at the seaside, in a rainforest or near a running waterfall is that the air in such natural places is super-charged with negative ions. These are tasteless, odourless and invisible molecules in environments like mountains, beaches and forests believed to raise the mood-chemical serotonin.

Conversely, it's also believed that one of the reasons we can feel more stressed in cities, air-conditioned environments, around computers or in more polluted areas is that the air in such environments is said to be charged with *positive* ions, which might increase stress, tension and tiredness.[18]

~~~~~~~~~

GET OUTSIDE

Vitamin D deficiency is becoming endemic in people who work long hours and see little light. Research is now showing that adequate levels are essential to both mood- and weight-management, as well as bone health and cancer-prevention.[19] The best source for humans is UV light on the skin.[20]

If you can't get outside to work out, spend 10 minutes outside in direct sunlight (without sunscreen), exposing your face and forearms, or 30 minutes when it's dull or cloudy. We need this every day for healthy vitamin D levels and you need longer exposure the darker your skin.

At the UK's University of Essex, researchers have extensively studied the wellbeing effects of outdoor exercise and have found that three-quarters of outdoor exercisers tested felt less angry, depressed or tense, compared with only half of those who worked out in a gym. Plus, the same team has also found that only five minutes spent in nature can have a positive impact on mood.[21]

We have a synergy with green plants: they oxygenate us while using our waste gas carbon dioxide for their own energy production. We breathe more deeply in the countryside and so relax our face, shoulders and mind, whereas in the face of pollution we protect ourselves with more shallow breathing and upper body tension. Exercising outside while being exposed to natural light has also been shown to help alleviate the symptoms of depression,[22] balance hormones such as melatonin and cortisol to help sleep/wake cycles and prevent the onset of Seasonal Affective Disorder (seasonal winter depression). One study found that women who walked outside experienced far more elevations in mood afterwards than those who walked inside.[23]

Being outside in the fresh air also increases the thermogenic effects of exercise. This means that the more you recondition yourself to exercise and live in slightly colder conditions, the more you reset your body to burn fat rather than store it.

Warm-up

A good warm-up prepares your body for exercise, helps prevent injury and can allow you time to consciously connect to your body's needs today. Walking is one of the best ways to ease the body into increasing blood flow to the working muscles and stimulate natural joint lubrication. Here are some other options:

At home:

- March on the spot for five minutes
- Walk up and down stairs for five minutes
- Walk or walk/jog around the park/block for 10 minutes

At the gym:

- Ten minutes easy pace on the cardio machine of your choice
- Ask a class instructor of any type if you can participate in his or her warm-up and afterwards, quietly leave the class to continue your own workout in another part of the gym – a good instructor shouldn't mind if you do this.

QUICK STRENGTH TRAINING

Studies have shown that people who do shorter, high-intensity toning exercise lose more fat and weight (especially around the middle)[24] and maintain more stable blood sugar than those doing traditional aerobic exercise for hours on end.[25] Lightweight training is one of the best ways of increasing muscle tone, but it doesn't have to be on bulky machines. It can incorporate light weights or even your own body as the force, as many yoga poses do.

A cleverly designed programme can follow muscle patterns that our ancestors would have used and that move intelligently through the body as it was designed; this approach is often referred to as *Primal Movement*.

If you're a gym member you can talk to a personal trainer about this type of workout and there are now classes available. At www.charlottewattshealth.com you'll find a free ebook of the De-Stress Strength Training Routine from Charlene Hutsebaut to do at home, in a park or at the gym. This covers an all-body intelligent toning of press-ups, wall squats with bicep curls, double arm rows, lunges, bridge pose and oblique abdominal rollbacks.

Benefits of lightweight training

The single biggest factor influencing your metabolism is the amount of muscle in your body. This is not about bulky biceps or hamstrings but sleek, long muscles that come from smart – not hard – exercise. For years, exercise junkies were obsessed with that magic 'calories burned' number on the treadmill as the Holy Grail of fat loss.

But more and more exercise physiologists are realizing that not only is this long, hard slog exhausting and highly stressful for the body, it's also the least important or beneficial way to work out. What matters is your caloric *afterburn*, the amount you burn *after* your workout. This is determined by the amount of muscle tone in your body. The right workout can elevate your Resting Metabolic Rate (RMR) for longer. This is optimized by activities that maximize muscle toning and *excess post-exercise oxygen consumption* (EPOC) – in other words, caloric afterburn.[26]

For gym bunnies

Shorter, higher-intensity workouts that increase EPOC are done for 30 minutes maximum. These can include circuit training, interval training and short, intense anaerobic exercises, such as sprints, with less intense recovery periods. Recovery time can be 24 to 48 hours, so alternating days with low-intensity movement like yoga, Pilates, walking and swimming is key to fitness as beneficial stress.

Cool-down

Don't simply spring up out of any exercise and leave in a flurry of stress. Spend a minute or two stretching muscles and relaxing; see the information on flexibility on page 201 and do yoga poses 14, 4, 5, 6 (raise arms and lean to each side), 13 and 15 for a targeted sequence (and another at www.charlottewattshealth.com).

Stretching adequately after exercise helps muscles recover more quickly and prevent post-workout muscle soreness.[27] By lengthening connective tissues, muscles and ligaments, the body's range of movement is kept mobile to reduce the likelihood and severity of injuries both from exercise and everyday life, including stress tension.[28]

ACTIVE REST

In his book *The Power of Rest: why sleep alone is not enough*, Dr Matthew Edlund talks about the four types of *active* rest our bodies need.[29] Sleep and watching TV are both types of passive rest, but most essential to rewiring and renewing our bodies are other forms of active rest for deep inner and outer renewal of our minds and bodies. Here are the doctor's four types of essential active rest:

Physical rest

Physical rest is an active, deliberate form of relaxation in which you use your body's basic physical processes, such as breathing, to calm and restore your body and mind. The mindful breathing, restorative yoga and guided relaxations explained in chapters 15 and 17 are these types of rest, as would be a 15–20 minute maximum daytime nap (see page 150).

Social rest

Human beings evolved as social beings, which is why we need to connect with friends we trust and whose company we enjoy to truly recharge and fortify ourselves. A huge bank of studies has shown that the one factor that differentiates happy people from not so happy souls is the power of their connections with others. Social withdrawal is a key sign of low serotonin, whereas social interaction releases beta-endorphins to help break the vicious cycle.

Social rest can be making a special one-to-one connection with someone you care about, visiting a neighbour or co-worker you would like to get to know better, making quick, healthy social connections (selective Facebook and Twitter communications), and going for a walk and a chat with a friend in the park. Laughter is a crucial component. Whether it's a phone call with someone who can see the funny side of life, stand-up comedy, movies or bad jokes, if you do nothing else to De-Stress, find something or someone that makes you chortle and feel good about yourself.

Mental rest

While in physical rest, you use your body's physical processes to calm and restore. In mental rest, the mind focuses to reach the meditative 'alpha' brainwave state where we can mentally rejuvenate. Any mindful or yoga practice can have this effect when we reach a level of complete absorption.[30]

Listen to your body

Learn the difference between being simply demotivated and actually needing to rest.

You need to rest or keep your exercise gentle if you:

- Feel heavy and lethargic morning after morning upon waking

- Have a feeling of having 'heavy legs' day after day

- When trying a light workout, feel that this strong fatigue or 'heavy legs' still exists

- Feel exhausted after exercise

You're demotivated and might benefit from a workout if you:

- Fantasize about lying on the sofa instead of doing something active or sociable

- Feel working out is 'too hard'

- Can come up with detailed excuses to convince yourself that it's a bad idea

- Attempt exercise and after about 10 minutes feel a renewed sense of energy – if you don't feel refreshed after exercise you need more rest

Help for your specific Stress Suit

All types can benefit from the strength training at www.charlottewattshealth. com, with the following specific exercise considerations taken into account:

Best exercise by Stress Suit	
Stressed and Wired	Slow down, even if you've become addicted to the hard workout. Recovery is crucial as you learn to relax. If you're a jogger, do walk/jog sessions with light jogging to lessen the risk of overtraining. Also try walking, Pilates and swimming. Stay away from hard, steady, long cardiovascular activities.
Stressed and Tired/ Stressed and Cold	Outdoor walks/activities for fresh air, with time to breathe and come out of 'daytime fog'. Schedule workouts/activities during the day if possible so that energy has had time to build up. Don't force evening workouts as these can tire you out more.
Stressed and Bloated	Try Pilates or yoga postures in seated, all fours or standing positions, with neutral back to encourage belly connection. Outdoor walks or activities in the fresh air increase abdominal circulation. Leave two to three hours after eating before exercising.

(continued)

Best exercise by Stress Suit	
Stressed and Sore	If you have sore or painful joints, avoid impact activities with bouncing, jumping or landing. Weight training strengthens bones and maintains healthy joint lubrication. Avoid long, hard cardiovascular workouts and choose walk/jogs or walking instead. Watch stress levels closely to avoid setting off inflammatory responses. Hydrate well so inflammatory histamines are less likely to be produced in the body after exercise.
Stressed and Demotivated	Opt for group activities for socialization, such as gentle yoga, dancing and other low-intensity classes. Morning workouts can help to increase feelings of vitality and mood, especially in the winter months. Buddy/ friend workouts help motivate you to attend, and add a social aspect to lift mood.
Stressed and Hormonal	Opt for group classes for support and socialization. Move every day – exercise is crucial for hormone balance through circulation and detoxification. Walking at times of your period or sugar cravings can decrease pain and take your mind off cravings.

Epilogue

A Cherokee proverb tells of an old man who said to his grandson: 'There is a battle between two wolves inside us all. One is Evil. It is anger, jealousy, greed, resentment, inferiority, lies and ego. The other is Good. It is joy, peace, love, hope, humility, kindness, empathy and truth.' The boy thought about this and then asked his grandfather, 'Which wolf wins?' The old Cherokee replied simply, 'The one you feed.'

Congratulations on reaching this point! Now is a great time to take stock and record what works best for you and what doesn't. What feeds your stressy habits and which routes back to De-Stress work for you?

Practice: The De-Stress reflection journal

Below is a reflective practice that will help form the basis of a personal De-Stress journal. You can keep coming back to your response to the questions here, to help you reflect on how your De-Stress lifestyle is making you feel and function, and to identify any tweaks you need to make.

1. Are you feeling more connected to your body and intuition around food, stress and your day-to-day needs?

2. Have you identified where you might tend to 'push on through', despite your body's obvious cries for rest, care and support?

3. Are sweet foods tasting too sweet? Are you enjoying the more subtle tastes of good-quality produce and flavourings?

4. Note how different days require different approaches. Are you now learning to be adaptable and to respect your body's altering needs, rather than expecting one strategy to work every single day?

5. Have you noticed any particular eating/energy patterns over three- or four-day cycles?

6. Variety is key, so don't settle into new fixed regimens – our ancestors ate hundreds more foods than we do and these changed with the seasons, limiting the likelihood of food intolerance and providing the right nutrient balance for the climate. Have you found ways to vary your food content to ensure your shopping and cooking are rewarding and done mindfully rather than on auto-pilot?

7. Have you assessed your relationship with grains and beans – will it work best for you to include some occasionally or are you feeling so good that you want to continue mainly to avoid them?

8. Too much of anything – partying, working, parenting – without the requisite balance of recharging and self-care will always wear you down. Are there any areas of your life where you still see yourself creating unnecessary stress? What kind of limits could you place on yourself to free yourself up for other pursuits that calm or energize you – for example, watching less TV in order to read more?

9. Has the way you cope with stress changed? Think about any habitual reactions, such as overeating, sugar cravings or flying off the handle, that you might have experienced when stress hit before you began the plan. When was the last time this happened, and how did you cope?

10. Are you managing to bring breathing techniques, mindfulness and movement into your life to help relieve stress on a daily basis? Which of these work best for you? A few minutes is all it takes.

11. Do you feel you've started on a journey and may need further investigation with a nutritional therapist or naturopath for food intolerance, thyroid function or adrenal stress testing? If the symptoms listed in the Stress Suits chapter still feel entrenched you may need to seek out more specific attention.

This is the beginning of a deeper journey with yourself and your needs; hopefully one that will spill out into positive effects throughout your whole life. Any change you make – even one – can set a ripple effect in motion that feeds into more. The following resources are available to you for help on my website www.charlottewattshealth.com:

- Register for the De-Stress Effect email support programme during your six-week plan, and to download the Progress Charts below

- Sign up for my weekly newsletter and receive free extras: meditation, body scan and yoga nidra audios; De-Stress Supplement Guide; De-Stress Strength Training and De-Stress Eating 7-Day Meal Plan ebooks.

- Downloads for extra help: The Stress Gauge, Reflection Journal, Monitoring Change and Classic Food Diary, so you can create a file for your personal preferences

- De-Stress Yoga Sequences and Strength Training Workout videos; more audios and videos

- More food suggestions and recipes

- Nutrition, yoga, mindfulness and self-care articles archive

- Information on webinars, workshops, classes and retreats

- Case studies to illustrate that you're not alone!

- A glossary to help you navigate terms used in the book

The De-Stress Effect Progress Charts
When you sign up at my website, you'll have access to a folder of charts designed to help you explore a new stress-free flow:

1. Daily Living Chart – a complete picture of a De-Stress day to help you focus on which habits to change at any time

2. What to Eat – an overview of De-Stress Eating to help guide change

3. Changing Your Food Habits – for noting down what might need changing and at a level you decide

4. Mood, Energy, Appetite – helping you to work out which foods and lifestyle choices make you feel best and will suit your health and weight-loss goals long term

5. Alcohol Intake Chart – this will help you get an overview of your drinking habits and make the best choices

Use the Progress Charts for:

- learning and memory tools as you start out

- help in deciding your levels of progressive change and noting how they made you feel

- guides to help you get back should you have an off-day

- reflective diaries for charting what suits you long term

- occasional 'check-ins' to take the 'stress temperature' of your life.

I have been on a long and fascinating journey to really delve into what makes me tick and how to stay connected to that in this crazy world. I truly hope this books helps you navigate life's rich pageant with a little more calm, easy and joy…

Good luck and enjoy exploring!

Charlotte x

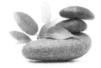

References

Chapter 1: Is Stress Ruling Your Life, Health and Happiness?

1. Stress at Work – Facts and Figures. European Agency for Safety and Health at Work. European Risk Observatory Report 2009

2. Reay G., Iddon B. Report by All Party Parliamentary Drugs Misuse Group: Inquiry into Physical Dependence and Addiction to Prescription and Over-the-Counter Drugs. 2008–2009

3. Skillsoft Report: Research into UK Workers' Stress Levels, online survey 2008, accessed August 2011

4. Epel E.S. et al. Stress and body shape: stress-induced cortisol secretion is consistently greater among women with central fat. Psychosom Med. 2000;62(5):623–32

5. Epel E.S. et al. Stress may add bite to appetite in women: a laboratory study of stress-induced cortisol and eating behavior. Psychoneuroendocrinology. 2001;26(1):37–49

6. Epel E.S. et al. Stress and body shape: stress-induced cortisol secretion is consistently greater among women with central fat. Psychosomatic Medicine. 2000;62:623–632

7. Park A. Fat Bellied Monkeys Suggest Why Stress Sucks. Time Magazine. August 8, 2009

8. Debigare R. et al. Catabolic/Anabolic Balance and Muscle Wasting in Patients with COPD. Chest. 2003;124(1):83–89

9. Falconer I.R. et al. Effect of adrenal hormones on thyroid secretion and thyroid hormones on adrenal secretion in the sheep. J Physiol. 1975;250(2):261–273

10. Block J.P. et al. Psychosocial Stress and Change in Weight Among US Adults. Am. J. Epidemiol. 2009;170(2):181–192

11. Tian R. et al. A possible change process of inflammatory cytokines in the prolonged chronic stress and its ultimate implications for health. Scientific World Journal. 2014 published online ahead of print

12. Klarer M et al. Gut vagal afferents differentially modulate innate anxiety and learned fear. J Neurosci. 2014;34(21):7067–76

13. Kakiashvili T. et al. The medical perspective on burnout. Int J Occup Med Environ Health. 2013;26(3):401–12

14. Ruttle P.L. et al. Disentangling psychobiological mechanisms underlying internalizing and externalizing behaviors in youth: Longitudinal and concurrent associations with cortisol. Hormones and Behavior. 2011;59(1):123

15. Chida Y., Steptoe A. Cortisol awakening response and psychosocial factors: a systematic review and meta-analysis. Biol Psychol. 2009;80(3):265–78

16. Papadopoulos A.S. Hypothalamic-pituitary-adrenal axis dysfunction in chronic fatigue syndrome. Nat Rev Endocrinol. 2011;8(1):22–32

Chapter 2: De-Stress for Improved Quality of Life

1. Shamantha Project: http://mindbrain.ucdavis.edu/labs/Saron/lab-news/The%20Shamatha%20Project.pdf accessed October 2014

2. Kemeny M.E. et al. Contemplative/emotion training reduces negative emotional behavior and promotes prosocial responses. Emotion. 2012;12(2):338–50

Chapter 3: Enjoy Each Moment

1. Smeets E. et al. Meeting suffering with kindness: effects of a brief self-compassion intervention for female college students. J Clin Psychol. 2014;70(9):794–807

Chapter 4: How Stress Creates Loops

1. Gallup A.C., Gallup G.G. Jr. Yawning and thermoregulation. PhysiolBehav. 2008;95(1–2):10–6.

2. Vlemincx E. Sigh rate and respiratory variability during mental load and sustained attention. Psychophysiology. 2011; 48(1):117–120

3. Mattson M.P. Hormesis Defined. Ageing Res. Rev. 2008;7(1):1–7

4. Dr Mark Mattson in interview with Anna Magee, quoted with kind permission

5. Aschbacher K. et al. Good stress, bad stress and oxidative stress: insights from anticipatory cortisol reactivity. Psychoneuroendocrinology. 2013;38(9):1698–708

6. Sun X. et al. Effects of mental resilience on neuroendocrine hormones level changes induced by sleep deprivation in servicemen. Endocrine. 2014 [Epub ahead of print]

7. Huether G. et al. The stress-reaction process and the adaptive modification and reorganization of neuronal networks. Psychiatry Research.1999;87(1):83–957

8. Hoge E.A. Loving-Kindness Meditation practice associated with longer telomeres in women. Brain Behav Immun. 2013;32:159–63

9. Gragnoli C. Hypothesis of the neuroendocrine cortisol pathway gene role in the comorbidity of depression, type 2 diabetes, and metabolic syndrome. Appl Clin Genet. 2014;7:43–53

10. Hostinar C.E., Gunnar M.R. Future directions in the study of social relationships as regulators of the HPA axis across development. J Clin Child Adolesc Psychol. 2013;42(4):564–75

11. Ditzen B., Heinrichs M. Psychobiology of social support: the social dimension of stress buffering. Restor Neurol Neurosci. 2014;32(1):149–62

Chapter 5: Which Stress Suit Are You Wearing?

1. Kyrou I. et al. Stress, visceral obesity, and metabolic complications. Ann NY Acad Sci. 2006;1083:77–110.

2. McEwan B. Protective and damaging effects of stress mediators. NEJM. 1998;338(3):171–179

3. What is Functional Medicine? The Institute for Functional Medicine www.functionalmedicine.org/What_is_Functional_Medicine/AboutFM/ accessed October 2014

4. Weatherby D. Signs and Symptoms Analysis from a Functional Perspective. Weatherby & Associates, LLC; 2nd edition 2004

5. Pizzorno J.E., Murray M.T. Textbook of Natural Medicine. Churchill Livingstone; 3rd edition 2010

6. Pruessner J.C. et al. Burnout, perceived stress, and cortisol responses to awakening. Psychosom Med. 1999;61(2):197–204

7. Anderson D.C. Assessment and nutraceutical management of stress-induced adrenal dysfunction. Integrative Medicine. 2008;7(5)

8. Mohler H. GABAA Receptors in Central Nervous System Disease: Anxiety, Epilepsy, and Insomnia. Journal of Receptors and Signal Transduction. 2006;26(5–6):731–740

9. Wilson J. Adrenal Fatigue, the 21st-Century Stress Syndrome. Smart Publications 2002

10. Ko F.N. et al. Vasodilatory action mechanisms of apigenin isolated from Apiumgraveolens in rat thoracic aorta. BiochimBiophysActa. 199;1115(1):69–74

11. Murck H. Magnesium and affective disorders. NutrNeurosci. 2002;5(6):375–89

12. Cernak I. et al. Alterations in magnesium and oxidative status during chronic emotional stress. Magnes Res. 2000;13(1):29–36

13. Seelig M.S. Consequences of magnesium deficiency on the enhancement of stress reactions; preventive and therapeutic implications (a review). Journal of the American College of Nutrition. 1994;13(5) 429–446

14. Galan P. et al. Dietary magnesium intake in a French adult population. Magnesium Research. 1997;10(4):321–328

15. Quaranta S. et al. Pilot study of the efficacy and safety of a modified-release magnesium 250 mg tablet (Sincromag) for the treatment of premenstrual syndrome. Clin Drug Investig. 2007;27(1):51–8

16. Fries E. et al. A new view on hypocortisolism. Psychoneuroendocrinology. 2005;30(10):1010–6.

17. Miller G.E. et al. If it goes up, must it come down? Chronic stress and the hypothalamic-pituitary-adrenocortical axis in humans. Psychol Bull. 2007;133(1):25–45

18. Heim C. et al. The potential role of hypocortisolism in the pathophysiology of stress–related bodily disorders. Psychoneuroendocrinology. 2000;25(1):1–35

19. Oelkers W. Adrenal insufficiency. NEJM;335 (16):1206–1212

20. Scherrer U., Sartori, C. Insulin as a vascular and sympathoexcitatory hormone. Circulation.1997;96:4104–4113

21. Progression of Stages of Adrenal Exhaustion. BioHealth Diagnostics. 2004;55

22. Swain M.G., et al. Fatigue in Chronic disease. Clinical Science. 2000;99:1–8

23. Neustadt J. Mitochondrial dysfunction and disease. Integrative Medicine. 2006;5(3)

24. Norris J., Messina G. B12 in Tempeh, Seaweeds, Organic Produce, and Other Plant Foods.

25. Charmandari E. et al. Pediatric stress: hormonal mediators and human development. Horm Res. 2003;59(4):161–79

26. SaitGonen M. et al. Assessment of anxiety in subclinical thyroid disorders. Endocrine Journal. 2004;51(3):311–5

27. Durrant-Peatfield B. Adrenal and Thyroid Gland Testing and Protocols. Lecture Notes attended Genova Diagnostics 2005

28. Son H.Y. et al. Synergistic interaction between excess caffeine and deficient iodine on the promotion of thyroid carcinogenesis in rats pretreated with N-bis(2-hydroxypropyl) nitrosamine. Cancer Sci. 2003;94(4):334–7

29. Vanderpas J. Nutritional epidemiology and thyroid hormone metabolism. Annu. Rev. Nutr. 2006;26: 293–322

30. Verhoeven D.T. et al. A review of mechanisms underlying anticarcinogenicity by brassica vegetables. Chem. Biol. Interact. 1997;103(2):79–129

31. Triggiani V. et al. Role of iodine, selenium and other micronutrients in thyroid function and disorders. EndocrMetab Immune Disord Drug Targets. 2009;9(3):277

32. Brzozowska M. et al. Evaluation of influence of selenium, copper, zinc and iron concentrations on thyroid gland size in school children with normal ioduria. Pol MerkurLekarski. 2006;20(120):672–7

33. Collins S.M., Bercik P. The relationship between intestinal microbiota and the central nervous system in normal gastrointestinal function and disease. Gastroenterology. 2009;136(6): 2003–14

34. Lyte M. et al. Induction of anxiety-like behavior in mice during the initial stages of infection with the agent of murine colonic hyperplasia Citrobacter rodentium. PhysiolBehav. 2006;30;89(3):350–7

35. Knowles S.R. et al. Investigating the role of perceived stress on bacterial flora activity and salivary cortisol secretion: a possible mechanism underlying susceptibility to illness. BiolPsychol 2008;77(2):132–7

36. Hawrelak J.A., Myers S.P. The causes of intestinal dysbiosis: a review. Altern Med Rev. 2004;9(2):180–97

37. Lutgendorff F. et al. The role of microbiota and probiotics in stress-induced gastro-intestinal damage. CurrMol Med. 2008;8(4):282–98

38. Ash M. A Novel Approach to Treating Depression – How Probiotics Can Shift Mood by Modulating Cytokines. Nutri-Link Ltd – Clinical Education. 2009

39. Kirkham M., Martin S. Eat less, chew more: getting the basics right for successful treatment. CAM. 2005:26–31

40. Hughes C. Galactooligosaccharide supplementation reduces stress-induced gastrointestinal dysfunction and days of cold or flu: a randomized, double-blind, controlled trial in healthy university students. Am J ClinNutr. 2011;93(6):1305–1311

41. Parnell J.A. Weight loss during oligofructose supplementation is associated with decreased ghrelin and increased peptide YY in overweight and obese adults. Am J ClinNutr. 2009;89(6):1751–1759

42. Francis C.Y. Bran and irritable bowel syndrome: time for reappraisal. The Lancet. 1994;344(8914):39–40

43. Drago S. Gliadin, zonulin and gut permeability: Effects on celiac and non-celiac intestinal mucosa and intestinal cell lines. Scandinavian Journal of Gastroenterology. 2006;41(4):408–419

44. Dolfini E. Damaging effects of gliadin on three-dimensional cell culture model. World J Gastroenterol. 2005;11(3):5973–77

45. Auricchio S. et al. Gluten-sensitive enteropathy in childhood. PediatrClin North Am. 1988;35(1):157–87

46. Jönsson T. et al. Agrarian diet and diseases of affluence – Do evolutionary novel dietary lectins cause leptin resistance? BMC Endocrine Disorders. 2005;5:10

47. Dixit V, Mak T.W. NF-kappa B signalling. Many roads lead to Madrid. Cell 2002;111:615–619

48. Lee D.F., Hung M.C. All roads lead to m-TOR: integrating inflammation and tumor angiogenesis. Cell Cycle 2007;6:3011–3014

49. Harbuz M. et al. Hypothalamo-pituitary-adrenal axis and chronic immune activation. Ann NY Acad Sci.2003;992, 99–106

50. Padgett D.A., Glaser R. How stress influences the immune response. Trends Immunol. 2003;24(8):444–8

51. Epel E.S. et al. Accelerated telomere shortening in response to life stress. ProcNatlAcadSci USA. 2004;101(49):17312–5

52. Harbuz M. et al. Hypothalamo-pituitary-adrenal axis and chronic immune activation. Ann NY Acad Sci. 2003;992:99–106

53. Khaustova S.A. et al. Short highly intense exercise causes changes in salivary concentrations of hydrocortisone and secretory IgA. Bull Exp Biol. 2010;149(5):635–9

54. Elenkov I.J., Chrousos G.P. Stress, cytokine patterns and susceptibility to disease. ClinEndocrinolMetab. 1999;13(4):583–95

55. Sivamani R. et al. Stress-mediated increases in systemic and local epinephrine impair skin wound healing: Potential new indication for beta blockers. PLoS, 2009;6(1):e12

56. Raison C.L. et al. Interferon-alpha effects on diurnal hypothalamic-pituitary-adrenal axis activity: relationship with proinflammatory cytokines and behavior. Mol Psychiatry. 2010;15(5):535–47

57. Robels T.F. et al. Out of Balance: A New Look at Chronic Stress, Depression, and Immunity. Current Directions in Psychological Science. 2005;14(2):111–115

58. Melpomeni P. et al. Glucose, Advanced Glycation End Products, and Diabetes Complications: What Is New and What Works. Clinical Diabetes. 2003;21(4):186–187

59. Simopoulos A.P. The Mediterranean Diets: What Is So Special about the Diet of Greece? The Scientific Evidence. J. Nutr. 2001;131:3065S–3073S

60. Freed D.L.F. Do dietary lectins cause disease? The evidence is suggestive – and raises interesting possibilities for treatment. BMJ. 1999;318(7190):1023–1024

61. Gupta Y.P. Antinutritional and toxic factors in food legumes: a review. Plant Foods for Human Nutrition.1987;37:201–228

62. James M. et al. Fish oil and rheumatoid arthritis: past, present and future. ProcNutr Soc. 2010;69:316–323

63. Wall R. et al. Fatty acids from fish: the anti-inflammatory potential of long-chain fatty acids. Nutr Rev. 2010;68:280–289

64. Leonard B.E. The HPA and immune axes in stress: the involvement of the serotonergic system. Eur Psychiatry. 2005;20:S302–6

65. Rada P. et al. Daily bingeing on sugar repeatedly releases dopamine in the accumbens shell. Neuroscience. 2005;134(3):737–44

66. Dallman M.F. Stress-induced obesity and the emotional nervous system. Trends EndocrinolMetab. 2010;21(3):159–165

67. Avena N.M. Examining the addictive-like properties of binge eating using an animal model of sugar dependence. ExpClinPsychopharmacol. 2007;15(5):481–91

68. Warne J.P. Shaping the stress response: interplay of palatable food choices, gluco-corticoids, insulin and abdominal obesity. Mol Cell Endocrinol. 2009;300(1–2):137–46

69. Shelton R.C, Miller A.H. Eating ourselves to death (and despair): the contribution of adiposity and inflammation to depression. ProgNeurobiol. 2010;91(4):275–99

70. Pecoraro N. et al. Chronic stress promotes palatable feeding, which reduces signs of stress: feedforward and feedback effects of chronic stress. Endocrinology. 2004;145(8):3754–62

71. Raison C.L. et al. Cytokines sing the blues: inflammation and the pathogenesis of depression.TrendsImmunol. 2006;27(1):24–31

72. Swenne I. Omega-3 polyunsaturated essential fatty acids are associated with depression in adolescents with eating disorders and weight loss. ActaPaediatr. 2011 [Epub ahead of print]

73. Office of Dietary Supplements. Dietary Supplement Fact Sheet: Vitamin D (Health Professional). US National Institutes of Health http://ods.od.nih.gov/factsheets/vitamind#h5 accessed October 2014

74. Walf A.A., Frye C.A. Review and Update of Mechanisms of Estrogen in the Hippocampus and Amygdala for Anxiety and Depression Behavior. Neuropsychopharmacology 2006;31:1097–1111

75. Textbook of Functional Medicine. Institute for Functional Medicine. 2005;19:229

76. Glenville M. Mastering Cortisol: Stop Your Body's Stress Hormone from Making You Fat Around the Middle. Amorata Press 2006

77. Touillaud M.S. et al. Dietary lignan intake and postmenopausal breast cancer risk by oestrogen and progesterone receptor status. J Natl Cancer Inst. 2007;99(6):475–867

78. Shu X.O. et al. Soy food intake and breast cancer survival. JAMA. 2009; 302(22):2437–43

79. Liener I.E. Implications of antinutritional components in soybean foods. Crit Rev Food SciNutr. 1994;34:31–67

80. Gold E.B. et al. Diet and lifestyle associated with premenstrual symptoms in a racially diverse community sample: Study of Women's Health Across the Nation (SWAN).

81. J Womens Health. 2007;16(5):641–56

82. Kavlock R.J. et al. Research needs for the risk assessment of health and environmental effects of endocrine disruptors: A report of the U.S. EPA sponsored workshop. Environ. Health Perspect. 1996;104(4):715–740

83. Malekinejad H. et al. Naturally occurring oestrogens in processed milk and in raw milk (from gestated cows). J Agric Food Chem. 2006;54(26):9785–91

Chapter 6: De-Stress Eating Principles

1. Turner B.L., Thompson A.L. Beyond the Paleolithic prescription: incorporating diversity and flexibility in the study of human diet evolution. Nutr Rev. 2013;71(8):501–10

2. Chauveau P. et al. Evolution of the diet from the paleolithic to today: progress or regress? Nephrol Ther. 2013;9(4):202–8

3. Carrera-Bastos P. et al. The Western diet and lifestyle and diseases of civilization. Res Rep ClinCardiol 2011;2:215–235

4. Chahwan R. The Multidimensional Nature of Epigenetic Information and Its Role in Disease. Discov Med. 2011(58):233–243

5. Frassetto L.A. et al. Metabolic and physiologic improvements from consuming a paleolithic, hunter-gatherer type diet. Eur J ClinNutr 2009;63(8):947–55

6. O'Keefe J.H. et al. Achieving hunter-gatherer fitness in the 21st century: back to the future. Am J Med. 2010;123(12):1082–6

7. Johnson J.B. et al. The effect on health of alternate day calorie restriction: eating less and more than needed on alternate days prolongs life. Med Hypothese. 2006;67(2):209–11

8. Cordain L. The nutritional characteristics of a contemporary diet based upon Paleolithic food groups. J Am Nutraceut Assoc. 2002;5:15–24

9. Henderson L. et al. The National Diet and Nutrition Survey: adults aged 19 to 64 years. Volume 3: Vitamin and Mineral intake and urinary analytes. TSO (London 2003)

10. Jönsson T. et al. Beneficial effects of a Paleolithic diet on cardiovascular risk factors in type 2 diabetes: a randomized cross-over pilot study. CardiovascDiabetol. 2009;8:35

11. Simopoulos A.P. The Mediterranean Diets: What Is So Special about the Diet of Greece? The Scientific Evidence. J. Nutr. 2001;131:3065S–3073S

12. O'Dea K. Marked improvement in carbohydrate and lipid metabolism in diabetic Australian aborigines after temporary reversion to traditional lifestyle. Diabetes. 1984;33(6):596–603

13. Osterdahl M. et al. Effects of a short-term intervention with a paleolithic diet in healthy volunteers. Eur J ClinNutr. 2008;62(5):682–685

14. Lieberman D., The Story of the Human Body: Evolution, Health and Disease. Penguin 2014 p.173

15. Simopoulos A.P. The Mediterranean Diets: What Is So Special about the Diet of Greece? The Scientific Evidence. J. Nutr. 2001;131:3065S–3073S

16. Lieberman D., The Story of the Human Body: Evolution, Health and Disease. Penguin 2014 p.91

17. Frank B.H. Are refined carbohydrates worse than saturated fat? Am J ClinNutr. 2010;91(6):1541–1542

18. Hite A.H. et al. In the face of contradictory evidence: Report of the Dietary Guidelines for Americans Committee. Nutrition. 2010;26(10):915–924

19. Yin X. et al. Ghrelin fluctuation, what determines its production? Acta Biochim Biophys Sin. 2009;41(3):188–197

20. Feinma R.D. 'A calorie is a calorie' violates the second law of thermodynamics. Nutr J. 2004;3:9

21. Larsen T.M. et al. Diets with high or low protein content and glycemic index for weight-loss maintenance. N Engl J Med. 2010;363(22):2102–13

22. Halton T.L. et al. The Effects of High Protein Diets on Thermogenesis, Satiety and Weight Loss: A Critical Review. J Am CollNutr. 2004;23(5):373–385

23. Vinknes K.J. et al. Dietary Intake of Protein Is Positively Associated with Percent Body Fat in Middle-Aged and Older Adults. J. Nutr. 2011;141(3):440–446

24. O'Dea K. Marked improvement in carbohydrate and lipid metabolism in diabetic Australian aborigines after temporary reversion to traditional lifestyle. Diabetes 1984;33(6):596–603

25. O'Dea K. Westernisation, insulin resistance and diabetes in Australian aborigines. Med J Aust. 1991;155(4):258–64

26. Daniel M. et al. Diabetes incidence in an Australian aboriginal population: an 8-year follow-up study. Diabetes Care.1999;22:1993–1998

27. Lindeberg S. et al. Cardiovascular risk factors in a Melanesian population apparently free from stroke and ischaemic heart disease: the Kitava study. J Intern Med. 1994;236:331–340

28. Lieberman D., The Story of the Human Body: Evolution, Health and Disease. Penguin 2014 p.224

29. Gannon M.C., Nuttall F.Q. Control of blood glucose in type 2 diabetes without weight loss by modification of diet composition. Nutrition & Metabolism 2006;3:16

30. Avena N.M. Examining the addictive-like properties of binge eating using an animal model of sugar dependence. ExpClinPsychopharmacol. 2007;15(5):481–91

31. Dallman M.F. Stress-induced obesity and the emotional nervous system. Trends EndocrinolMetab. 2010;21(3):159–165

32. Lindgärde F. Traditional versus agricultural lifestyle among Shuar women of the Ecuadorian Amazon: effects on leptin levels. Metabolism. 2004;53(10):1355–8

33. Lieberman D., The Story of the Human Body: Evolution, Health and Disease. Penguin 2014 p.103

34. Hite A.H. Low-Carbohydrate Diet Review: Shifting the Paradigm. NutrClinPract. June 2011;26(3):300–308

35. Kristen G. et al. Lifestyle Factors and 5-Year Abdominal Fat Accumulation in a Minority Cohort: The IRAS Family Study. Obesity. 2011;171

36. Freed D.L.J. Do dietary lectins cause disease? The evidence is suggestive – and raises interesting possibilities for treatment. BMJ. 1999;318(7190):1023–1024

37. Jönsson T. et al. Agrarian diet and diseases of affluence – Do evolutionary novel dietary lectins cause leptin resistance? BMC Endocrine Disorders. 2005;5:10

38. Ruales J. Saponins, phytic acid, tannins and protease inhibitors in quinoa (Chenopodiumquinoa, Willd) seeds. Food Chemistry. 1993;48(2)137–143

39. Macfarlane B.J. et al. Inhibitory effect of nuts on iron absorption. Am J ClinNutr. 1988 Feb;47(2):270–4

40. Tuntawiroon M. Rice and iron absorption in man. Eur J ClinNutr. 1990;44(7):489–97

41. Kelsay J.L. A review of research on effects of fiber intake on man. Am J ClinNutr. 1978;31(1):142–159

42. Reddy N.R. et al. Food Phytates. CRC Press 2001

43. Reinhold J.G. et al. Decreased Absorption of Calcium, Magnesium, Zinc and Phosphorus by Humans due to Increased Fiber and Phosphorus Consumption as Wheat Bread. J. Nutr. 1976;106(4):493–503

44. Famularo G. et al. Probiotic lactobacilli: an innovative tool to correct the malabsorption syndrome of vegetarians?. Med. Hypotheses. 2005;65(6):1132–5

45. Hemalatha S. et al. Influence of germination and fermentation on bioaccessibility of zinc and iron from food grains. Eur J ClinNutr. 2007;61(3):342–8

46. German J.B., Dillard C.J. Saturated fats: what dietary intake? Am J ClinNutr. 2004;80(3)550–559

47. Howard BV et al. Low-fat dietary pattern and risk of cardiovascular disease: the Women's Health Initiative Randomized Controlled Dietary Modification Trial. JAMA. 2006;295(6):655–66

48. Micha R, Mozaffarian D. Saturated fat and cardiometabolic risk factors, coronary heart disease, stroke, and diabetes: a fresh look at the evidence. Lipids. 2010;45(10):893–905

49. Ramsden C.E. et al. Dietary fat quality and coronary heart disease prevention: a unified theory based on evolutionary, historical, global, and modern perspectives. Curr Treat Options Cardiovasc Med. 2009;11(4):289–301

50. Mozaffarian D. et al. Effects on coronary heart disease of increasing polyunsaturated fat in place of saturated fat: a systematic review and meta-analysis of randomized controlled trials. PLoS Med. 2010;23;7(3):e1000252

51. Cordain L. et al. Plant-animal subsistence ratios and macronutrient energy estimations in worldwide hunter-gatherer diets. Am J ClinNutr. 2000;71(3):682–92

52. Cordain L et al. The paradoxical nature of hunter-gatherer diets: meat-based, yet non-atherogenic. Eur J ClinNutr. 2002;56(1):S42–52

53. Li Z et al. Dietary Factors Alter Hepatic Innate Immune System in Mice with Non-Alcoholic Fatty Liver Disease. Hepatology. 2005

54. Cordain L et al. Plant-animal subsistence ratios and macronutrient energy estimations in worldwide hunter-gatherer diets. Am J ClinNutr. 2000;71(3):682–92

55. Micallef M. et al. Plasma n-3 Polyunsaturated Fatty Acids are negatively associated with obesity. Br J Nutr. 2009;102(9):1370–4

56. McCombie G. et al. Omega-3 oil intake during weight loss in obese women results in remodelling of plasma triglyceride and fatty acids. Metabolomics. 2009;5(3):363–374

57. Parra D. et al. A diet rich in long chain omega-3 fatty acids modulates satiety in overweight and obese volunteers during weight loss. Appetite. 2008;51(3):676–80

58. Piscitelli F. et al. Effect of dietary krill oil supplementation on the endocannabinoidome of metabolically relevant tissues from high-fat-fed mice. NutrMetab. 2011;8(1):51

59. Kuipers R.S. et al. Estimated macronutrient and fatty acid intakes from an East African Paleolithic diet. Br J Nutr. 2010;104(11):1666–87

60. Lieberman D., The Story of the Human Body: Evolution, Health and Disease. Penguin 2014 p.224

61. Siri-Tarino P.W. et al. Meta-analysis of prospective cohort studies evaluating the association of saturated fat with cardiovascular disease. Am J ClinNutr. January 2010;ajcn.27725

62. Papamandjaris A.A. et al. Medium chain fatty acid metabolism and energy expenditure: obesity treatment implications. Life Sci. 1998;62(14):1203–15

63. Mañé J. et al. Partial replacement of dietary (n-6) fatty acids with medium-chain triglycerides decreases the incidence of spontaneous colitis in interleukin-10-deficient mice. J Nutr. 2009;139(3):603–10

64. Huang C.B. et al. Short- and medium-chain fatty acids exhibit antimicrobial activity for oral microorganisms. Arch Oral Biol. 2011;56(7):650–4

65. Thormar H. et al. Stable concentrated emulsions of the 1-monoglyceride of capric acid (monocaprin) with microbicidal activities against the food-borne bacteria Campylobacter jejuni, Salmonella spp., and Escherichia coli. Appl Environ Microbiol. 2006;72(1):522–6

66. Batovska D.I. et al. Antibacterial study of the medium chain fatty acids and their 1-monoglycerides: individual effects and synergistic relationships. Pol J Microbiol. 2009;58(1):43–7

67. Hauenschild A. et al. Successful treatment of severe hypertriglyceridemia with a formula diet rich in omega-3 fatty acids and medium-chain triglycerides. Ann NutrMetab. 2010;56(3):170–5

68. Nagao K., Yanagita T. Medium-chain fatty acids: functional lipids for the prevention and treatment of the metabolic syndrome. Pharmacol Res. 2010;61(3):208–12

69. St-Onge M.P. et al. Medium chain triglyceride oil consumption as part of a weight loss diet does not lead to an adverse metabolic profile when compared to olive oil. J Am CollNutr. 2008;27(5):547–52

70. Hite A.H. et al. In the face of contradictory evidence: Report of the Dietary Guidelines for Americans Committee. Nutrition. 2010;26(10):915–924

71. Pribila B.A. et al. Improved lactose digestion and intolerance among African-American adolescent girls fed a dairy-rich diet. J Am Diet Assoc. 2000;100(5):524–8

72. Tuula et al. Lactose Intolerance. Journal of the American College of Nutrition. 2000;19:165S-175S

73. Itan, Y. et al. The Origins of Lactase Persistence in Europe. PLoS Computational Biology. 2009;5(8): e1000491

74. Hoppe C. et al. High intakes of milk, but not meat, increase s-insulin and insulin resistance in 8-year-old boys. Eur J ClinNutr. 200;59(3):393–8

75. Bulhoes, A.C. et al. Correlation between lactose absorption and the C/T-13910 and G/A-22018 mutations of the lactase-phlorizin hydrolase (LCT) gene in adult-type hypolactasia. Brazilian Journal of Medical and Biological Research. 2007;11

76. Anderson D.C. Assessment and nutraceutical management of stress-induced adrenal dysfunction. Integrative Medicine. 2008;7(5)

77. Aschoff J. et al. Meal timing in humans during isolation without time cues. J Biol Rhythms.1986;1(2):151–62

78. Cugini P. et al. Chronobiometric identification of disorders of hunger sensation in essential obesity: therapeutic effects of dexfenfluramine. Metabolism. 1995;44(2):50–6

Chapter 7: Understanding Cravings

1. Weingarten H.P. et al. Food cravings in a college population. Appetite. 1991;17:167–175
2. Rada P. et al. Daily bingeing on sugar repeatedly releases dopamine in the accumbens shell. Neuroscience. 2005;134(3):737–44
3. Groesz L. et al. What is eating you? Stress and the Drive to Eat. Appetite 2012;58(2): 717–721
4. Pecina S. et al. Nucleus accumbenscorticotropin-releasing factor increases cue-triggered motivation for sucrose reward: paradoxical positive incentive effects in stress? BMC Biology 2006;4:8
5. Erlanson-Albertsson C. Sugar triggers our reward-system. Sweets release opiates which stimulates the appetite for sucrose – insulin can depress it. Lakartidningen. 2005;102(21):1620–2
6. Blass E. et al. Interactions between sucrose, pain and isolation distress. PharmacolBiochem Behav.1987;26(3):483–9
7. Warne J.P. Shaping the stress response: interplay of palatable food choices, glucocorticoids, insulin and abdominal obesity. Mol Cell Endocrinol. 2009;300(1–2):137–46
8. Deckersbach et al. Pilot randomized trial demonstrating reversal of obesity-related abnormalities in reward system responsivity to food cues with a behavioral intervention. Nutrition & Diabetes 2014, published online
9. Adam T.C. et al. Stress, eating and the reward system. Physiology & Behaviour. 2007;91(4):449–458
10. Krebs H. et al. Effects of stressful noise on eating and non-eating behavior in rats. Appetite.1996;26(2):193–202
11. Wang G. et al. Gastric stimulation in obese subjects activates the hippocampus and other regions involved in brain reward circuitry. Proceedings of the National Academy of Science. 2006;103(42)15641–15645
12. García-Cáceres C., Tschop M.H. The emerging neurobiology of calorie addiction. eLife Published online Jan 2014 10.7554/eLife.01928
13. Hoebel B.G. et al. Evidence for sugar addiction: Behavioral and neurochemical effects of intermittent, excessive sugar intake. Neuroscience and Biobehavioral Reviews. 2008;32:20–39
14. Baumeister R.F. et al. The Strength Model of Self Control. Current Directions in Psychological Science. 2007;16
15. Fritz Strack et al. Reflective and Impulsive Determinants of Social Behaviour. Personality and Social Psychology. Review 2004
16. Alberts H.J. et al. Dealing with problematic eating behaviour. The effects of a mindfulness-based intervention on eating behaviour, food cravings, dichotomous thinking and body image concern. Appetite 2012;58(3):847–51
17. Beshara M. et al. Does mindfulness matter? Everyday mindfulness, mindful eating and self-reported serving size of energy dense foods among a sample of South Australian adults. Appetite 2013;67:25–9
18. Rogojanski J. et al. Role of sensitivity to anxiety symptoms in responsiveness to mindfulness versus suppression strategies for coping with smoking cravings. J Clin Psychol. 2011;67(4):439–45

19. Lacaille J. et al. The effects of three mindfulness skills on chocolate cravings. Appetite 2014;76:101–12

Chapter 8: De-Stress Eating Basics

1. Uematsu T. et al. Effect of dietary fat content on oral bioavailability of menatetrenone in humans. J Pharm Sci. 1996;85(9):1012–6

2. Shin J.S. et al. Indole-Containing Fractions of Brassica rapa Inhibit Inducible Nitric Oxide Synthase and Pro-Inflammatory Cytokine Expression by Inactivating Nuclear Factor-κB. J Med Food. 2011 [Epub ahead of print]

3. Karen-Ng L.P. et al. Combined Effects of Isothiocyanate Intake, Glutathione s-Transferase Polymorphisms and Risk Habits for Age of Oral Squamous Cell Carcinoma Development. Asian Pac J Cancer Prev. 2011;12(5):1161–6

4. Bulhões A.C. et al. Correlation between lactose absorption and the C/T-13910 and G/A-22018 mutations of the lactase-phlorizin hydrolase (LCT) gene in adult-type hypolactasia. Braz J Med Biol Res. 2007;40(11):1441–1446

5. deVrese M. et al. Probiotics – compensation for lactase insufficiency. Am. J. Clin. Nutr. 2001;73 (2): 421S–429S

6. Ho S. et al. Comparative effects of A1 versus A2 beta-casein on gastrointestinal measures: a blinded randomised cross-over pilot study. Eur J Clin Nutr. 2014;68(9):994–1000

7. Kamiński S. et al. Polymorphism of bovine beta-casein and its potential effect on human health. J Appl Genet. 2007;48(3):189–98

Chapter 9: Six Weeks to De-Stress Eating

1. Ifland J.R. et al. Refined food addiction: a classic substance use disorder. Med Hypotheses. 2009;72(5):518–26

2. Ledochowski M. et al. Fructose malabsorption is associated with decreased plasma tryptophan. Scand. J. Gastroenterol. 2001;36 (4):367–71

3. Stanhope K.L. Adverse metabolic effects of dietary fructose: results from the recent epidemiological, clinical, and mechanistic studies. Curr Opin Lipidol. 2013;24(3):198–206

4. Fernandes et al. Mouse study: Aspartame consumption in diabetes-prone mice. The University of Texas Health Science Center San Antonio 2011 http://www.uthscsa.edu/hscnews/singleformat2.asp?newID=3861 accessed October 2014

5. Yang Q. Gain weight by 'going diet?' Artificial sweeteners and the neurobiology of sugar cravings. Yale J Biol Med. 2010;83(2):101–108

6. Wideman C.H. et al. Implications of an animal model of sugar addiction, withdrawal and relapse for human health. NutrNeurosci. 2005 ;8(5–6):269–76

7. http://education.wichita.edu/caduceus/examples/soda/tbspn_in_can.html accessed October 2014

8. Amo K. et al. Effects of xylitol on metabolic parameters and visceral fat accumulation. J ClinBiochemNutr. 2011;49(1):1–7

9. Jarvill-Taylor K.J. et al. A hydroxychalcone derived from cinnamon functions as a mimetic for insulin in 3T3-L1 adipocytes. J Am CollNutr. 2001 Aug;20(4):327–36

10. Bocarsly M.E. et al. Rats that binge eat fat-rich food do not show somatic signs or anxiety associated with opiate-like withdrawal: Implications for nutrient-specific food addiction behaviors. PhysiolBehav. 2011 [Epub ahead of print]

11. Tylka T.L. Development and psychometric evaluation of a measure of intuitive eating. Journal of Counseling Psychology. 2006;53(2):226–240

12. Hairston et al. Lifestyle Factors and 5-Year Abdominal Fat Accumulation in a Minority Cohort: The IRAS Family Study. Obesity 2012;20(2):421–7

13. Hemalatha S. et al. Influence of germination and fermentation on bioaccessibility of zinc and iron from food grains. Eur J ClinNutr. 2007;61(3):342–8

14. Di Cagno R. et al. Proteolysis by sourdough lactic acid bacteria: effects on wheat flour protein fractions and gliadin peptides involved in human cereal intolerance. Appl Environ Microbiol. 2002;68:623–633

15. Avena N.M., Hoebel B.G. A diet promoting sugar dependency causes behavioral cross-sensitization to a low dose of amphetamine. Neuroscience. 2003;122(1):17–20

16. Blum K. et al. Dopamine and glucose, obesity, and reward deficiency syndrome. Front Psychol. 2014;5:919

Chapter 10: The Building Blocks of Healthy Eating

1. Duckett S.K. Understanding Factors Affecting Meat Quality – Results from Pasture Based Beef Systems – 3 year multi State Study. American Grassfed Association. 2007

2. Micha R. et al. Red and processed meat consumption and risk of incident coronary heart disease, stroke, and diabetes mellitus: a systematic review and meta-analysis. Circulation. 2010 Jun 1;121(21):2271–83

3. EDF Seafood Selector. Environmental Defense Fund. http://seafood.edf.org/guide/ accessed October 2014

4. Williams D.E. et al. Xenobiotics and xenoestrogens in fish: modulation of cytochrome P450 and carcinogenesis. Mutation Research/Fundamental and Molecular Mechanisms of Mutagenesis. 1998;399(2):179–192

5. Kastel M.A. Maintaining the Integrity of Organic Milk. The Cornucopia Institute. Presented to the USDA National Organic Standards Board 2006

6. Butler G. et al. Fat composition of organic and conventional retail milk in northeast England. J Dairy Sci. 2011;94(1):24–36

7. C.J. Puotinen. Unhealthy Vegetable Oils? Does Food Industry Ignore Science Regarding Polyunsaturated Oils? Implications for Cancer, Heart Disease. Well Being Journal. 2005;14(3)

8. Block E. The Chemistry of Garlic and Onion. Sci Am 1985;252:94–99

9. Layrisse M. et al. New property of vitamin A and B carotene on human iron absorption: effect on phytate and polyphenols as inhibitors of iron

10. Hemalatha S. et al. Influence of heat processing on the bioaccessibility of zinc and iron from cereals and pulses consumed in India. J Trace Elem Med Biol. 2007;21(1):1–7

11. Gautam S. et al. Higher bioaccessibility of iron and zinc from food grains in the presence of garlic and onion. J Agric Food Chem. 2010;58(14):8426–9

12. Gautam S. et al. Influence of combinations of promoter and inhibitor on the bioaccessibility of iron and zinc from food grains. Int J Food SciNutr. 2011 [Epub ahead of print]

13. Nachbar et al. Lectins in the United States diet: a survey of lectins in commonly consumed foods and a review of the literature. Am J Clin Nutr. 1980;33(11) 2338–2345

Chapter 11: A Morning Revolution

1. Timlin M.T. Breakfast Eating and Weight Change in a 5-Year Prospective Analysis of Adolescents: Project EAT (Eating Among Teens). Pediatrics. 2008;3:e638–e645

2. Rampersaud G.C. et al. Breakfast habits, nutritional status, body weight, and academic performance in children and adolescents.. J Am Diet Assoc. 2005;105(5):743–60

3. Blom W.A.M. et al. Effect of a high-protein breakfast on the postprandial ghrelin response. Am J ClinNutr 2006;83(2):211–220

4. Kapur et al. Postprandial Insulin and Triglycerides after Different Breakfast Meal Challenges: Use of Finger Stick Capillary Dried Blood Spots to Study Postprandial Dysmetabolism. J Diabetes Sci Technol. 2010;4(2):236–243

5. Tin S.P. et al. Breakfast skipping and change in body mass index in young children. Int J Obes. 2011;35(7):899–906

6. Dhurandhar N.V. et al. Egg breakfast enhances weight loss. FASEB J. 2007;21:538

7. Vander Wal J.S. et al. Egg breakfast enhances weight loss. Int J Obes. 2008;32(10):1545–51

8. Ratliff J. et al. Consuming eggs for breakfast influences plasma glucose and ghrelin, while reducing energy intake during the next 24 hours in adult men. Nutr Res. 2010;30(2):96–103

9. Pal S., Lim S. The effect of a low glycaemic index breakfast on blood glucose, insulin, lipid profiles, blood pressure, body weight, body composition and satiety in obese and overweight individuals: a pilot study. J Am CollNutr. 2008;27(3):387–93

10. Isaksson H. et al. Effect of rye bread breakfasts on subjective hunger and satiety: a randomized controlled trial. Nutr J. 2009 Aug 26;8:39

Chapter 12: Recharging Daytime

1. Research carried out in 2009 by Spar

2. Diekelmann S. and Born J. The memory function of sleep. Nature Reviews Neuroscience 2010;11:114–126

Chapter 13: Mindful Evenings

1. Head K., Kelly G. Nutrients and botanicals for treatment of stress: Adrenal fatigue, neurotransmitter imbalance, anxiety, and restless sleep. Alt. Med. Rev. 2009;14(2):114–140

2. Backhaus J. et al. Sleep disturbances are correlated with decreased morning awakening salivary cortisol. Psychoneuroendocrinology. 2004;29 (9): 184–91

3. Moss T.G. et al. Is daily routine important for sleep? An Investigation of social rhythms in a clinical insomnia population. Chronobiol Int. 2014:1–11. [Epub ahead of print]

4. Yang X. A wheel of time: the circadian clock, nuclear receptors, and physiology. Genes Dev. 2010;24:741–747

5. Shang Y. et al. Imaging analysis of clock neurons reveals light buffers the wake-promoting effect of dopamine. Nat Neurosci. 2011;14(7):889–95

6. Sole M.J. et al. Diurnal physiology: core principles with application to the pathogenesis, diagnosis, prevention, and treatment of myocardial hypertrophy and failure. Journal of Applied Physiology. 2009;107(4):1318–1327

7. Mustian K.M. Multicenter, randomized controlled trial of yoga for sleep quality among cancer survivors. J Clin Oncol. 2013;10;31(26):3233–41

8. Halpern J. et al. Yoga for improving sleep quality and quality of life for older adults. Altern Ther Health Med. 2014;20(3):37–46

9. Holt S.H.A. et al, A Satiety Index of Common Foods. European Journal of Clinical Nutrition. 1995:675–690

10. Winkelman J.W. Reduced Brain GABA in Primary Insomnia: Preliminary Data from 4T Proton Magnetic Resonance Spectroscopy (1H-MRS). Sleep. 2008;31(11):1499–1506

11. Abdou A.M. et al. Relaxation and immunity enhancement effects of gamma-aminobutyric acid (GABA) administration in humans. Biofactors. 2006;26(3):201–8

12. Cheng S.T. et al. Improving Mental Health in Health Care Practitioners: Randomized Controlled Trial of a Gratitude Intervention. J Consult Clin Psychol. 2014 [Epub ahead of print]

Chapter 14: Stress-Free Drinks and Snacks

1. Duffey K.J., Popkin B.M. Energy Density, Portion Size, and Eating Occasions: Contributions to Increased Energy Intake in the United States, 1977–2006. PLoS Med 2011;8(6)

2. Blom W.A.M et al. Effect of a high-protein breakfast on the postprandial ghrelin response. Am J ClinNutr 2006;83(2):211–220

3. Hazuda H.P. Human study: The San Antonio Longitudinal Study of Aging. The University of Texas Health Science Center San Antonio 2011

4. Francesco S. et al. Taste perception and implicit attitude toward sweet related to body mass index and soft drink supplementation. Appetite 2011

5. http://www.ipsos-mori.com/researchpublications/researcharchive/1982/Chocolate-Pushes-Sex-Into-Second-Place.aspx accessed October 2014

6. Buitrago-Lopez A. et al. Chocolate consumption and cardiometabolic disorders: systematic review and meta-analysis. BMJ. 2011;343:d4488

7. Drewnowski A. et al. Taste responses and preferences for sweet high-fat foods: evidence for opioid involvement. PhysiolBehav 1992;51(2):371–9.

8. Martin F.P. et al. Metabolic Effects of Dark Chocolate Consumption on Energy, Gut Microbiota, and Stress-Related Metabolism in Free-Living Subjects. J. Proteome Res 2009; 8(12):5568–5579

9. Tey S.L. et al. Nuts improve diet quality compared to other energy-dense snacks while maintaining body weight. J NutrMetab. 2011:357350

10. Cassady B.A. et al. Mastication of almonds: effects of lipid bioaccessibility, appetite and hormone response. Am J. Clin Nutr. 2009;89:794–800

11. McCartney. Waterlogged? BMJ 2011;343:d4280.

12. Saat M. et al. Rehydration after exercise with fresh young coconut water, carbohydrate-electrolyte beverage and plain water. J PhysiolAnthropolAppl Human Sci. 2002;21(2):93–104

13. O'Keefe J.H., Cordain L. Cardiovascular Disease Resulting From a Diet and Lifestyle at Odds With Our Paleolithic Genome: How to Become a 21st-Century Hunter-Gatherer. Mayo Clin Proc. 2004;79:101–10

14. Anderson D.C. Assessment and nutraceutical management of stress–induced adrenal dysfunction. Integrative Medicine. 2008;7(5)

15. Armstrong L.E. Caffeine, Body Fluid-Electrolyte Balance, and Exercise Performance. International Journal of Sport Nutrition & Exercise Metabolism. 2002

16. Psychol. 2010 Dec;85(3):496–8.

17. Amin N. et al. Genome-wide association analysis of coffee drinking suggests association with CYP1A1/CYP1A2 and NRCAM. Mol Psychiatry 2012;17(11):1116–29

18. Al-Qarawi A. et al. Liquorice (Glycyrrhizaglabra) and the adrenal-kidney-pituitary axis in rats. Food Chem2002;40(10):1525–1527

19. Hammer F., Stewart P.M. Cortisol metabolism in hypertension. Best Pract Res ClinEndocrinolMetab. 2006;20(3):337–53

20. Yang C.S., Wang H. Mechanistic issues concerning cancer prevention by tea catechins. Mol Nutr Food Res. 2011;55(6):819–31

21. Park K.S. et al. Epigallocatethin-3-O-gallate counteracts caffeine-induced hyperactivity: evidence of dopaminergic blockade. BehavPharmacol. 2010 Sep;21(5–6):572–5.

22. Higashiyama A. et al. Effects of l-theanine on attention and reaction time response. Journal of Functional Foods. 2011;3(3):171–178

23. Kim S. et al. Resveratrol exerts anti-obesity effects via mechanisms involving down-regulation of adipogenic and inflammatory processes in mice. BiochemPharmacol. 2011;81(11):1343–51

24. Simopoulos A.P. The Mediterranean Diets: What Is So Special about the Diet of Greece? The Scientific Evidence. J. Nutr. 2001;131:3065S–3073S

25. Cargiulo T. Understanding the health impact of alcohol dependence. American Journal of Health-System Pharmacy. 2007;64(5,3): S5–S11

26. Oscar-Berman M., Marinkovic K. Alcoholic Brain Damage. Alcohol Research & Health. 2003;27(2):125–133

27. Spreckelmeyer K.N. Opiate-Induced Dopamine Release Is Modulated by Severity of Alcohol Dependence: An [(18)F]Fallypride Positron Emission Tomography Study. Biol Psychiatry. 2011;70(8):770–6

28. Mishra D., Chergui K. Ethanol inhibits excitatory neurotransmission in the nucleus accumbens of adolescent mice through GABA(A) and GABA(B) receptors. Addict Biol. 2013;18(4):605–13

Chapter 15: The Mindfulness Practices

1. Matta C. Can Meditation Lower Your Risk for Heart Disease? http://blogs.psychcentral.com/dbt/2011/07/can-meditation-lower-your-risk-for-heart-disease/ accessed October 2014

2. Davidson R.J., Lut A. Buddha's Brain: Neuroplasticity and Meditation. IEEE Signal Processing Magazine. 2007 Sep;172–6

3. Kaul P. Meditation acutely improves psychomotor vigilance, and may decrease sleep need Behavioral and Brain Functions.2010;6:47

4. David Creswell J. et al. Brief mindfulness meditation training alters psychological and neuroendocrine responses to social evaluative stress. Psychoneuroendocrinology 2014;44:1–12

5. Pidgeon A.M. Evaluating the effectiveness of enhancing resilience in human service professionals using a retreat-based Mindfulness with Metta Training Program: a randomised control trial. Psychol Health Med. 2014;19(3):355–64

6. Hoge E.A. et al. Randomized Controlled Trial of Mindfulness Meditation for Generalized Anxiety Disorder: Effects on Anxiety and Stress Reactivity. J Clin Psychiatry 2013;74(8): 786–792

7. Chen K.W. et al. Meditative Therapies for Reducing Anxiety: A Systematic Review and Meta-analysis of Randomized Controlled Trials. Depress Anxiety. 2012;29(7):545–562

8. Carlson L.E. et al. Mindfulness-based stress reduction in relation to quality of life, mood, symptoms of stress and levels of cortisol, dehydroepiandrosterone sulfate (DHEAS) and melatonin in breast and prostate cancer outpatients. Psychoneuroendocrinology 2004;29(4):448–74

9. Pace T.W.W. et al. Effect of Compassion Meditation on Neuroendocrine, Innate Immune and Behavioral Responses to Psychosocial Stress. Psychoneuroendocrinology 2009;34(1):87–98

10. van der Riet P. et al. Piloting a stress management and mindfulness program for undergraduate nursing students: Student feedback and lessons learned. Nurse Educ Today 2014 [Epub ahead of print]

11. Hamilton et al. Brief guided imagery and body scanning interventions reduce food cravings. Appetite 2013;71:158–62

12. Gard T. et al. Fluid intelligence and brain functional organization in aging yoga and meditation practitioners. Front Aging Neurosci. 2014;6:76

Chapter 16: Yoga as Awareness

1. Taspinar B. et al. A comparison of the effects of hatha yoga and resistance exercise on mental health and well-being in sedentary adults: a pilot study. Complement Ther Med. 2014;22(3):433–40

2. Bryan S. et al. The effects of yoga on psychosocial variables and exercise adherence: a randomized, controlled pilot study. Altern Ther Health Med. 2012;18(5):50–9

3. Streeter C.C. et al. Effects of yoga on the autonomic nervous system, gamma-aminobutyric-acid, and allostasis in epilepsy, depression, and post-traumatic stress disorder. Med Hypotheses. 2012;78(5):571–9

4. DeVries H.A. et al. Tranquilizer effect of exercise. American Journal of Physical Medicine. 1981;60:57–66

5. Kristal A.R. Yoga practice is associated with attenuated weight gain in healthy, middle-aged men and women. AlternTher Health Med. 2005;11(4):28–33

6. Telles S. et al. Short term health impact of a yoga and diet change program on obesity. Med SciMonit. 2010;16(1):CR35–40.

7. The Effects of T. Krishnamacharya Style Yoga Class on Body Image of Female College Students. Department of Kinesiology, California State University CA. Submitted for publication http://www.wellnessnexus.com/page8/page19/about-amy.html accessed October 2014

8. Wheeler A. The Effects of a University Yoga Class on Nutritional Habits of Students. 2011, Department of Kinesiology, California State University CA. Submitted for publication

9. Martin R. et al. The role of body awareness and mindfulness in the relationship between exercise and eating behavior. J Sport Exerc Psychol. 2013;35(6):655–60

10. Kamei T. et al. Decrease in serum cortisol during yoga exercise is correlated with alpha wave activation. Percept Mot Skills. 2000;90(3,1):1027–32

11. Wheeler A., Wilkin L. A Study of the Impact of Yoga Âsana on Perceived Stress, Heart Rate, and Breathing Rate. International Journal of Yoga Therapy. 2007;17:57–63

12. Parthasarathy S. et al. Effect of Integrated Yoga Module on Selected Psychological Variables among Women with Anxiety Problem. West Indian Med J. 2014;63(1):83–85

13. Field T. Yoga clinical research review. Complementary Therapies in Clinical Practice. 2010:1–8

14. Sivasankaran S. The Effect of a Six-Week Program of Yoga and Meditation on Brachial Artery Reactivity: Do Psychosocial Interventions Affect Vascular Tone? Clin. Cardiol. 2006;29,:393–398

15. Conti P.B. Assessment of the body posture of mouth-breathing children and adolescents. J Pediatr (Rio J). 2011;87(4):357–63

16. Conrad A. Psychophysiological effects of breathing instructions for stress management. ApplPsychophysiol Biofeedback. 2007;32(2):89–98

17. Wheeler A. An Analysis of Personality, Yoga Preferences and the Relaxation Response. Presented at the International Association of Yoga Therapy Sytar Conference, 2007, Los Angeles, CA

18. Kalyani B.G. et al. Neurohemodynamic correlates of 'OM' chanting: A pilot functional magnetic resonance imaging study. Int J Yoga. 2011;4(1):3–6

19. Rajesh S.K. et al. Effect of Bhramari Pranayama on response inhibition: Evidence from the stop signal task. Int. J Yoga 2014;7(2):138–141

Chapter 18: The New Mind–body Movement

1. Hassmen P. et al. Physical Exercise and psychological well-being: a population study in Finland. Preventative Medicine. 2000;30(1):17–25

2. Childs E., de Wit H. Regular exercise is associated with emotional resilience to acute stress in healthy adults. Front Physiol. 2014;5:161 online

3. McClellan S., Hamilton B. So Stressed. Simon & Schuster 2010

4. L. Cordain et al. Physical Activity, Energy Expenditure and Fitness: An Evolutionary Perspective. International Journal of Sports Medicine. 1998;19(5):328–35

5. Biddle S. et al. Physical Activity and Psychological Wellbeing. Routledge 2000

6. Tremblay M.S. et al. Incidental movement, lifestyle-embedded activity and sleep: new frontiers in physical activity assessment. Can J Public Health. 2007;98(2):S208–17

7. Jakicic J.M. et al. Effect of exercise on 24 month weight loss maintenance in overweight women. Archives of Internal Medicine. 2008;168(14):1550–9

8. Taylor A., Katomeri M. Walking reduces cue-elicited cigarette cravings and withdrawal symptoms, and delays ad libitum smoking. Nicotine Tob Res. 2007;9(11):1183–90

9. Tudor-Locke C. et al. How many steps/day are enough? Sports Medicine.2004;34(1):1–8

10. Boreham C.A.G. et al. Training effects of short bouts of stair climbing on cardiorespiratory fitness, blood lipids, and homocysteine in sedentary young women. British Journal of Sports Medicine. 2005;39(9):590–593

11. Boyd S., Eaton M.B. The Paleolithic Prescription: A Program of Diet & Exercise and a Design for Living. Harper Collins 1989

12. O'Keefe J. et al. Achieving Hunter-gatherer Fitness in the 21st Century: Back to the Future. Amer J Med. 2010;123(12):1082–6

13. Wilson M. et al. Diverse patterns of myocardial fibrosis in lifelong, veteran endurance athletes. J Appl Physiol. 2011;110(6):1622–6

14. Jeffrey R. et al. A Time Series Diary Study of Mood and Social Interaction. Motivation and Emotion. 1998;22

15. Hull E. et al. Effects of dance on physical and psychological wellbeing in older persons. Archives of Gerontology and Geriatrics. 2009;49(1):e45–50

16. Hall S.A. et al. Sexual activity, erectile dysfunction and incident cardiovascular events. American Journal of Cardiology. 2010;105(2):192–7

17. Ebrahim S. et al. Sexual intercourse and risk or ischaemic stroke and coronary heart disease: the Caerphilly study. Journal of Epidemiological Community Health. 2002;56(2):99–102

18. Goldenberg M. et al. Why Individuals Hike the Appalachian Trail: A Qualitative Approach to Benefits. Journal of Experiential Education. 2008;30(3):277–281

19. Hideo N. et al. Effect of negative air ions on computer operation, anxiety and salivary chromogranin A-like immunoreactivity. IntJournPsychophys. 2002;46:85–89

20. Ramagopalan S.V. et al. A ChIP-seq defined genome-wide map of vitamin D receptor binding: Associations with disease and evolution. Genome Research. 2010;20

21. Holick M.F. The Vitamin D Epidemic and its Health Consequences. J Nutr. 2005;135:2739S–2748S

22. Pretty J. et al. A Countryside for Health and Well-Being: The Physical and Mental Health Benefits of Green Exercise. Report for the Countryside Recreation Network, February 20

23. Sami L. et al. Drop-out and mood improvement: a randomised controlled trial with light exposure and physical exercise. BMC Psychiatry. 2004;4:22

24. Teas J. et al. Walking Outside Improves Mood for Healthy Postmenopausal Women Oncology. 2007;1:35–43

25. Boutcher S.H. High Intensity Intermittent Exercise and Fat Loss. J Obes. 2011:865305

26. Trapp E.G. et al. The effects of high intensity intermittent exercise training on fat loss and fasting insulin levels of young women. International Journal of Obesity. 2008;32(4):684–91

27. DeVries H.A. et al. EMG comparison of single doses of exercise and meprobamate as to effects of muscular relaxation. American Journal of Physical Medicine. 1972;51:130–141

28. Bach B. et al. A comparison of muscular tightness in runners and non-runners and the relation of muscular tightness to low back pain in runners. Journal of Orthopedic Sports Physical Therapy. 1985;6:315–323

29. Edlund M. The Power of Rest: Why Sleep Alone Is Not Enough. A 30-Day Plan to Reset Your Body. HarperOne 2011. Quoted with kind permission from the author

30. Martin R. et al. The role of body awareness and mindfulness in the relationship between exercise and eating behavior. J Sport Exerc Psychol. 2013;35(6):655–60

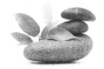

Bibliography

Anodea J., *Eastern Body, Western Mind: Psychology and the Chakra System as a Path to the Self* (Celestial Arts, 2004)

Baer R.A., *Mindfulness-based Treatment Approaches: A Clinician's Guide to Evidence Base and Approaches* (Academic Press, 2005)

Biddle, S. et al., *Physical Activity and Psychological Wellbeing* (Routledge, 2000).

Boyd, S., Eaton, M.B., *The Paleolithic Prescription: A Program of Diet & Exercise and a Design for Living* (Harper Collins, 1989)

Brach T., *True Refuge: Finding Peace and Freedom in Your Own Awakened Heart* (Hay House, 2013)

DesMaisons, K., *Potatoes Not Prozac* (Simon & Schuster, 2008)

Edlund, M., *The Power of Rest: Why sleep alone is not enough* (HarperCollins, 2010)

Farhi, D. *The Breathing Book: Vitality and Good Health Through Essential Breath Work* (Holt, 1996)

Glenville, M., *Mastering Cortisol: Stop Your Body's Stress Hormone from Making You Fat Around the Middle* (Amorata Press, 2006)

Hamilton D., *Why Kindness is Good for You* (Hay House, 2010)

Hanna T., *Somatics: Reawakening the Mind's Control of Movement, Flexibility, and Health* (Da Capo Press Inc, 2004)

Hanson R., *Buddha's Brain: The Practical Neuroscience of Happiness, Love, and Wisdom* (New Harbinger, 2009)

Kaminoff, L., *Yoga Anatomy: Your illustrated guide to postures, movements, and breathing techniques* (Human Kinetics Europe Ltd, 2007)

Kessler, D., *The End of Overeating: Taking control of our insatiable appetite* (Penguin, 2010)

Koch L., *Core Awareness, Revised Edition: Enhancing Yoga, Pilates, Exercise, and Dance* (North Atlantic Books, 2012)

Lasater J., *Living Your Yoga: Finding the Spiritual in Everyday Life* (Rodmell Press, 2000)

Lieberman D., *The Story of the Human Body: Evolution, Health and Disease* (Penguin, 2014)

Long, R., *Scientific Keys Volume I: The Key Muscles of Hatha Yoga* (3rd edn; Bandha Yoga, 2006)

Lucas M., *Rewire Your Brain for Love: Creating Vibrant Relationships Using the Science of Mindfulness* (Hay House, 2013)

McClellan, S., Hamilton, B., *So Stressed* (Simon & Schuster, 2010)

Pizzorno J.E., Murray M. T., *Textbook of Natural Medicine* (3rd edn; Churchill Livingstone, 2010)

Sapolsky, R.M., *Why Zebras Don't Get Ulcers* (Holt, 2004)

Smolensky, M., Lamberg, L., *The Body Clock Guide to Better Health* (Holt, 2000)

Stiles, M., *Structural Yoga Therapy: Adapting to the Individual* (Red Wheel/Weiser, 2000)

Wansink, J., *Mindless Eating* (Hay House, 2011)

Weatherby, D., *Signs and Symptoms Analysis from a Functional Perspective* (2nd edn; Weatherby & Associates, LLC, 2004)

Wilberg P., *Head, Heart and Hara: The Soul Centres of West and East* (New Gnosis Publications, 2003)

Wilson, J., *Adrenal Fatigue, the 21st-Century Stress Syndrome* (Smart Publications, 2002)

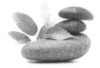

Acknowledgements

First and foremost, a deep-felt thank you to my friend and co-author on this book's first incarnation, *The De-Stress Diet*: the gorgeous, kind, funny and smart journalist and Healthista.com creator and editor, Anna Magee. Our journey together allowed me to move those ideas towards this book and our work together still forms its foundation.

Then, many thanks to the many pioneering and brilliant clinicians and scientists whose ground-breaking work has been quoted in this book, and whose ideas and vision have been instrumental in shaping *The De-Stress Effect*. Without their work, my research and understanding of nutrition, the nature of stress and the innate wisdom of mindfulness and yoga – and much more – would simply not have been possible.

To name a few: Marion Kirkham ND, Chris Astill-Smith, Dr Nigel Plummer, Dr Robert Verkerk, Dr Jeffrey Bland, Lyra Heller, Stephen Terass, Alessandro Ferretti, Roderick Lane, Thích Nhất Hạnh, Jon Kabat-Zinn, Tara Brach, Dr Rick Hanson, Dr Kristin Neff, Marsha Lucas PhD, Mariane Northrup, Thomas Hanna, Moshe Feldenkrais, Nutri-Link Education, Dr Mark Mattson, Dr Matthew Edlund, Dr Loren Cordain, Professor Robert Sapolsky, Dr Bart Hoebel and the Institute for Optimum Nutrition.

Special thanks go to the nurturers and supporters of my vision, most notably, the insightful and savvy Hay House team who shaped the wave that carried this book to fruition: Michelle Pilley, Amy Kiberd and Jo Burgess, along with the fabulous Julie Oughton. The whole process has only been wonderful, smooth and a beautiful example of mindful professionalism.

Debra Wolter's sensitive and skilful editing process followed suit to fine-tune and mould a finished product that makes me very happy. Also, massive thanks to Carolyn Thorne, who initially commissioned *The De-Stress Diet*. Her perseverance was essential to the existence of *The De-Stress Effect*.

This book would not have been possible without the exceptional input of trusted consultants. Fitness trainer Charlene Hutsebaut (charlenehutsebaut.com) brought her authority, experience and knowledge of modern movement, anatomy and fitness to Chapter 18, making it the effective package we hope it becomes for the reader.

Nutritional cooking consultant Tina Deubert has brought a wealth of food preparation knowledge, passion and instinct to the recipes and cooking advice in this book. All the illustrations are by the very talented Jackie Coulson, whose lovely yoga teaching shows in her drawing style. Gratitude also to Corinna Gordon-Barnes and Cheryl Richardson, for their invaluable and *heartful* business acumen and advice.

My life and work, both reflected deeply in this book, have been majorly influenced by my yoga and spiritual journey. My first yoga teacher, Jim Tarran, is owed special thanks for shaping the way I teach and practise. He allowed me to understand how to hold energy, intense sensation and my fractured self – even when this was extremely difficult – and much of my language and teaching empathy is rooted in this care.

Teachers since who have resonated profoundly and whose words are all channelled in this book are Cathy-Mae Karelse, David Lichfield and Lotus Nguyen for their rich teaching of mindfulness and the kind attention they embody; Judith Lasater for her wise, illuminating, joyous and explorative presence; Tias Little for the poetry he brings to anatomy and energetics – his skull-sacrum polarity work (and more) is referred to in chapter 16; and Donna Farhi for her fierce clarity and embodied teaching; her fluidity work and freedom to simply move and attend gracefully was invaluable.

A huge shout out to my beautiful friend and yoga buddy Khadine Morcom. Our discussions, laughter and stays in hotels exploring our yoga and mindfulness journey are woven into these pages and have been some of the most joyous times in my life.

Great thanks to the inimitable Heather Mason, whose campaigning to bring yoga and mindfulness into mainstream health care has provided me with some key ideas and research included here. Last, but certainly not least, gratitude to the lovely Fiona Agombar, whose yoga therapy and personal relationship with her practice has inspired me greatly.

Oodles of thanks to my dad ('Grandad') for always turning up to save the day and continually providing subversive merriment. Thanks too to Maisie's dad, Sam, for supporting the conscious process of this book's unfolding and for following its ethos with our daughter. Huge, cuddly love and thanks to my daughter, Maisie, for being a most excellent and inspirational source of 'good stress' and providing fun, fantastic chats, brilliant insights and constant hilarity.

Index

Index

~

ABOUT THE AUTHOR

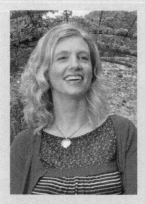

Charlotte Watts is a Nutritional Therapist who has been practising since 2000, winning the CAM Award for Outstanding Practice in 2012. She studied at The Institute of Optimum Nutrition, London, where she went on to become a second year tutor and Year 3 Programme Leader. She has since lectured for the College of Naturopathic Medicine and The Minded Institute. She is a regular speaker and was the co-presenter on the BBC3 series *Freaky Eaters*.

Charlotte has been practising yoga since 1996, studying to be a teacher at the Vajrasati School in Brighton (500 hours Yoga Alliance certified). She further trained in yoga as therapy for fatigue and stress states, and continues to study with teachers who combine her love of mindful, somatic practice and yoga as meditation. She trains teachers in Yoga for Stress and Burnout at Yoga Campus, London.

In over a decade of seeing clients privately, Charlotte has had great success in helping people become healthier, happier and feeling more in control of their lives. She firmly believes that we need to look at our lives as a whole to improve our health and quality of life, and has attracted many celebrity and high-profile clients. Charlotte is the author of *100 Top Recipes for Happy Kids*, *100 Best Foods for Pregnancy* and *100 Foods to Stay Young*. She features regularly in the UK press, has a monthly column in *Om* magazine and blogs weekly for healthista.com. She also runs classes, workshops and retreats.

Charlotte lives in Brighton in the southeast of England with her gorgeous daughter, Maisie.

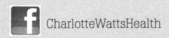 CharlotteWattsHealth   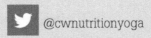 @cwnutritionyoga

www.charlottewattshealth.com